HERE

IN THE

MIDDLE

STORIES OF LOVE, LOSS, AND CONNECTION FROM THE ONES SANDWICHED IN BETWEEN

EDITED AND CURATED BY

CHRISTINE ORGAN AND JULIE JO SEVERSON

HERE
IN THE
MIDDLE

STORIES OF LOVE, LOSS, AND CONNECTION FROM THE ONES SANDWICHED IN BETWEEN

EDITED AND CURATED BY

CHRISTINE ORGAN AND JULIE JO SEVERSON

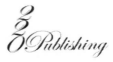

ADVANCE PRAISE FOR HERE IN THE MIDDLE

"The curators deftly meld individual writers' voices into a chorus of raw and honest stories. The authors' accounts of how they navigate precious and often complicated relationships will touch readers at any stage of life but will leave others in the sandwich generation feeling understood and connected."

~ **Caryn M. Sullivan**, Award-winning author of *Bitter or Better: Grappling With Life on the Op-Ed Page*, inspirational speaker and award-winning columnist

"This middle place – in between kids who are growing up too quickly and parents who look to us for help more than we look to them – is messy, confusing and overwhelming. This beautiful collection of essays will remind you that you're far from alone in the experience, and to treasure the days you have together with the people you love most. I'll revisit these pieces again and again!"

~ **Jill Smokler**, Founder of the parenting website, *Scary Mommy* and New York Times bestselling author

"*Here in the Middle* is a wonderful collection of essays that explores the uncertainty of middle age and everything that comes with it: love, loss, caregiving and the search for a strand of meaning to carry us through it all."

~ **Emily Gurnon**, Senior Content Editor, Health and Caregiving, PBS Next Avenue

"A glittering collection of stories for anyone struggling with life in the middle."

~ **Andra Watkins**, NY Times bestselling author of *Not Without My Father*

"The essays in *Here in the Middle* offer hope, understanding, compassion, and levity for anyone who is simultaneously caring for their children and aging parents. Christine Organ and Julie Jo Severson beautifully weave together stories that reflect on the evolving and sometimes confusing roles of child, then parent, and then... "*Here in the Middle*," where roles flip-flop, often without notice, leaving those in the middle feeling like they are "neither fully one place nor another," as one mother describes. Kudos to Christine and Julie for compiling this much-needed book, which provides sandwiched parents with a healthy dose of reality, strength, and comfort."

~ **Julie Burton**, Author of *The Self-Care Solution—A Modern Mother's Must-Have Guide to Health and Well-Being* (She Writes Press, 2016)

"*Here In The Middle* plucked at my heartstrings and brought tears to my eyes. Each essay resonated with me as a mom and as a daughter and reminded me that every relationship we fold ourselves into is a unique blessing to be cherished. These relationships are unconditional and everlasting, regardless of how life's pace waxes and wanes. This book can serve to teach something to those who haven't reached the middle quite yet, but for those of us who are there, *Here In The Middle* makes us feel somehow less alone."

~ **Dana Faletti**, author of *Beautiful Secret*

Published by 220 Publishing

(A Division of 220 Communications)

PO Box 8186

Chicago, IL 60680-8186

www.220communications.com

www.twitter.com/220comm

For more information on the authors, visit:

Christine Organ:

www.christineorgan.com

Julie Jo Severson:

www.carvingsonadesk.com

www.julieseverson.com

Cover and Interior Design by Christina Sanders

Cover image: © Billion Photos

ISBN 978-1-68419-780-4

Printed in USA

TABLE OF CONTENTS

AN INTRODUCTION TO THE MIDDLE
By Christine Organ

When I was nine years old, my grandpa—my mom's dad—was in a plane crash. He survived, but many people on the plane did not. The event was unsettling, to say the least, and I had several questions. But as most children do, I asked questions in search of reassurance and relativity to my own life. What caused the crash? Would Grandpa be okay? Is it safe to fly? Why don't all planes fall from the sky?

Over time, however, the crash receded into the backdrop of our family's life and eventually the questions subsided.

Until recently.

Lately I've been asking the questions again, wondering, looking at the situation through a more introspective, grown-up lens. Perhaps the natural progression of life leads us to wonder about death and recognize life's fragility. Or maybe it's because my oldest son is 9 years old—the same age I was when the crash happened—and I'm in that poignant middle place as both daughter and mother. Whatever the reason, some time ago, a few of the old questions returned, along with several new ones. What did my grandpa think in those terrifying moments of impact? How did my grandma react when she got the telephone call? And how did this catastrophe impact my own parents' marriage?

Even though I can no longer ask my grandpa these questions—he lived well into his 80s before succumbing to a brain tumor—I could ask my mom and my grandma about the crash and its aftermath on our family with a fair amount of comfort they'd provide the answers from which they'd protected me when I was a child.

But what I realize as I become further entrenched in this middle place—watching my parents get older, comforting friends whose parents have died, caring for friends my own age as they deal with cancer and other health nightmares, answering my kids' questions about death and God, and feeling days and years slip by in a flurry of homework assignments, doctor appointments, and work meetings—is that most of my questions about the plane crash are the ones that don't have any answers. I find myself asking the tough questions, the uncomfortable questions that in some fundamental way, seem oddly pertinent to my own life.

About a year ago, my mom and I went through old newspaper clippings salvaged from the days and weeks after my grandpa's plane crash. I was writing an essay on the experience and wanted to know more. We searched for answers and tried to understand more about what had happened and who had been affected. But given that the crash happened before the age of the Internet, the information was rather limited.

I wanted to know about the father who, I'd heard, took an earlier flight home to watch his son play in a Little League game. Was that true? Or was it something that I'd conjured in my mind as a child based on a snippet of information? And if it was true, what happened to that little boy? How had he recovered? What was his life like now? No one could remember these details, and of course, there was no information on this little boy and his widowed mother. It seemed that with each new detail revealed, new questions emerged.

For instance, I learned that my grandpa had maintained a friendship with two fellow survivors from different cities and states, but the nature of that friendship remains a mystery. Was it a relationship defined by Christmas cards and quick phone calls every few years? Or was there something deeper there, a bond that can only be forged when people walk through fire (in this case, literally) together?

We also learned that one of the deceased passengers was a man planning to play racquetball with a friend that night; another was a husband with a wife and two toddlers waiting for him at home. Who were they? Did they say "I love you" to their significant others one last time before they boarded the plane? Or were their last words rushed and tainted with the chores of daily life? And why weren't their lives spared? Why did my grandpa get to live and they didn't?

And what about the ones who were left behind? How did *they* survive? How did they wake up the next day and the day after that, knowing that life as they'd known it was gone, permanently altered? How did they go on?

My mother and I ended our investigation longing for more. We both ached for more information. We wanted to know, to understand, to fill the gaps in the stories and our memories.

When my parents were in that same middle place I'm in now, they seemed, to me, to know what they were doing. They made decisions, built up their lives, and raised their children. They answered questions and taught us right from wrong. They had it all together. They'd arrived. They were grown-ups. I assumed when I "grew up," I'd be the one answering questions instead of asking them.

But then, at some point, I began to feel like I was trudging through a multi-dimensional hall of mirrors, asking questions that had multiple angles and complex answers, or no answers at all. Within the span of eighteen months, one of my best friends was diagnosed with breast cancer, another friend lost her mother unexpectedly, and my dad was diagnosed with various life-altering medical conditions. Mortality suddenly didn't look so distant. Life felt more fragile than ever.

As I talked with friends and family members who were also muddling through the middle, a few common themes began to take shape: density, confusion, and poignancy.

These middle years are a study in contrasts—feeling scared and safe, uncertain and confident, confused and wise all at the same time. My childhood assumption that being a grown-up meant having all the answers clearly was a myth. Maybe it's okay to say "I don't know" and hold on to a little mystery. Maybe we can be both reckless and careful, rolling the dice and taking a few risks now and then, planning for the future and playing it safe at other times.

The stories in the chapters ahead provide a variety of perspectives from those who've been touched by the mystery, beauty, even the levity of the middle years and within the circle of life.

They don't seek to "fix" a situation or provide answers on what a person should or shouldn't do. Rather, they create a sense of camaraderie and give voice to the poignancy and confusion, tenderness and grief, connection and anxiety that many feel while sandwiched between generations and responsibilities. By asking the unanswerable questions and sharing our stories, we can celebrate life for the buoyant gift that it is.

Curating this collection of essays, along with Julie Jo Severson, was an honor and true labor of love. We're both grateful to all those who submitted their stories and opened their hearts. We hope this book is a lifeboat of sorts. May the words sustain and uplift us when the waves get rocky. May the camaraderie help us to accept ourselves and the murkiness of this phase of life. And may the stories honor the preciousness of this fragile human life.

After all, what is life if not a journey across a wild and magnificent sea?

Christine Organ—co-curator and co-editor of this book— is a freelance writer who lives in the Chicago area with her husband and two sons. She is a staff writer for Scary Mommy and a regular contributor to Babble. Her work has also been published online with the New York Times, Washington Post, *Huffington Post, Mamalode,* Redbook, Country Living, Good Housekeeping, *and Brain, Child Magazine, among others. She has also been published in print magazines, including* UU World. *She is the author of* Open Boxes: the gifts of living a full and connected life *(a collection of stories that will make you feel really freaking good), and a contributor to* I Just Want to Be Perfect *(the fourth book in the bestselling* I Just Want to Pee Alone *series). You can often find her eating cookie dough or wasting time on Facebook, Twitter, and Instagram. She writes at www.christineorgan.com.*

BEYOND DESCRIBE
By Julie Jo Severson

"I have a poem!" my mom announced as she woke up from a dream at around four o'clock one spring morning in 2004 while nudging my dad awake so she could dictate it to him.

Under normal circumstances, Mom would've quietly written the poem down herself. Like she used to. By that time, though, she'd been living with Parkinson's disease for sixteen years, and her arms and legs felt as though they were slowly being encased in cement. Or so I once read somewhere and have tried to imagine.

Dad, in a wrinkly T-shirt and boxer shorts with a head of tousled bed hair, did what any good husband would do. He turned on the bedside lamp, opened the nightstand drawer, pulled out a piece of scratch paper and pen, and said, "Okay, I'm ready."

His hands became hers, and together they preserved her poem in ink:

I saw them come

from far and wide

just to see our children

who were beautiful

beyond describe

and just as God

had willed them.

By Mom

(*Diane Louise Martinka*)

***

"What's the object lesson in this?" I hear TV show host Charlie Rose ask a commentator in a PBS replay.

I look up from my laptop screen and over at Mom sitting across from me in her motorized lift chair, a medical alert pendant draped around her neck by a thin, black cord. She's fallen asleep—the TV remote is on the swivel tray in front of her, along with a small dish of chocolates, a glass of water with a straw, a tube of lip balm, and a couple of rosaries.

Her baby soft face, now loosely framed with hair

touching her shoulder that's as white and wispy as a snow angel, is one of the most naturally beautiful I've ever seen. Other than a little blush from time to time, I've rarely seen her wear makeup. She radiates on her own. I remember once as a little girl, sitting at the end of my parents' bed watching her get ready for an evening out, thinking how pretty she was. She's as luminous now as she was then.

I wonder if she's dreaming. Maybe she's dreaming she and Dad are young, wide-eyed newlyweds again sailing on the Queen Elizabeth, waves cresting and lapping, cool sea spray splashing into her face, sounds of seagulls and creaking wood of the ship lulling her into a peaceful bliss.

Or maybe she's dreaming about the big swing inside the screened-in porch of her grandparents' lake home she once reminisced about to me. She said it was like a mattress suspended from the ceiling. During summer visits as a little girl, she'd often sleep on it with the canvas curtains rolled up all around the porch.

"Oh think of it—that fresh air!" she had said to me.

I wouldn't be surprised if she's dreaming a poem like she did while lying next to my father in the wee hours of that spring morning all those years ago. Reciting a poem has become nearly as difficult as writing one down, now nearly thirty years since the Parkinson's was first diagnosed. She knows what words she wants to say, but at times they're slightly out of reach, or it's tiring for her to project them loud enough for us to hear. I suspect, though, there are lots of poems still swirling around inside her.

Sitting here with my eyes rested upon her while she sleeps, I'm pulled toward a love and longing impossible to define—*beyond describe*, words from a mother's dream inscribed in a poem.

Our physical roles as mother and daughter have switched places; our deep-down emotional roles have not. When I lean in to kiss her cheek each time I stop in for my regular weekday visits, she still smiles and looks into my eyes like a mother searching for clues to her daughter's heart. And I still yearn, like a child, for her to instinctively know without me having to say.

I'm here for the day to give Dad a chance to get out of the house, run a few errands, attend a seminar, pick up "some parts" at Menards, maybe get a haircut, or putz on projects in the garage or office with peace of mind. "I leave you in good hands," he often says to Mom, as he bends over and they embrace before he entrusts her in my care.

I have a writing project due in a couple days so I sit, for a little while, at a cleared-off spot on their second-hand dining table buried in Dad's newspapers, dated issues of *National Geographic* and *Time* magazine, church bulletins, pharmacy receipts, Fleet Farm flyers, and free mailing labels from the Society of the Little Flower.

Earlier I spent a few hours cleaning the toilet and shower, sweeping floors, checking dates in the fridge, straightening piles, pausing to flip through a family photo album, doing a couple loads of laundry, making lunch, helping Mom transfer to the wheelchair for a trip to the bathroom, and sitting beside her massaging her lower back, listening to music, and helping with small tasks.

A voracious reader, sometimes she hands me a piece of paper on which her stiffened fingers tried their best to wrap themselves around a pen and write down the name of a book she'd heard about while listening to one of her NPR shows. I search for it on Amazon and download it to her Kindle. We haven't done this lately, though. The buttons and touchscreen are getting difficult to navigate; the text, even set on large print, is often too taxing to read.

Other times, she wants me to sift through her plastic bin of greeting cards, which Dad keeps stocked for her thanks to the local dollar store. At her request, I select cards for family members with birthdays coming up, according to a laminated list of dates she keeps on the shelf next to her chair. She never misses a birthday. She whispers a message for me to write in each card, and then I address, stuff, seal, and stamp the envelopes. We have a big family, including twenty-five grandkids, so we work on birthday cards together a lot.

Then for fun, I might show her pictures of my kids and Oscar (my dog) on my phone, posts from family members on Facebook, or random YouTube videos. She likes the funny ones the best. We all love when Mom laughs. Despite some decrease in facial expression, a common symptom in this advanced stage, her laugh is legendary in our family. It starts as a low ripple in the chest, works its way up, then bursts through as a red-nosed, shoulder-shaking, tears-streaming-down-face geyser. When it happens, you stand back, revel in her glee, make sure she comes out of it still breathing and intact, and love her even more.

While potential what-if scenarios stir quietly in our minds and hearts, Mom and Dad are determined to live out their lives in their own home on their own terms. Or at least as long as possible. It's not easy, and we worry, but they have good reasons, and so, that's the current plan.

Mom enjoys her solitude and, of course, wants to live as independently as she can with the man sparkling in her eyes—still tall and slender with hair as white as hers—while he serves her yogurt in a wine glass, peels her oranges, refills her candy dish, and places his strong, wrinkled hand on her soft, smooth cheek.

Dad, dealing with his share of health challenges, too, is a die-hard, do-it-yourself kind of guy. He constructs wheelchair thresholds out of plywood, whips up homemade soups out of leftovers, installs grab bars, researches accessible vans and tubs, and hard-wires strategically placed "help buttons" made out of recycled doorbells to play various melodies, such as "Joy to the World," whenever that clever, coy, hazel-eyed country girl—his bride for nearly sixty years—pushes one for assistance.

My siblings and I help as much as our parents and our lives allow. When Dad periodically lands himself in the hospital for some reason or another, at least a couple times a year it seems, equally needing special care and attention—we rally. We come together in a magnetic, high-velocity force and flurry of group e-mails and texts, coordinating our schedules, stepping out of our everyday orbits to ensure one of us is with Mom at all times while keeping Dad company, too.

Thank God for siblings. There are nine of us. Some near, some far. It *still* doesn't seem like enough in those times. Each of us feels the pull and squish in our hearts and in our lives in different ways, longing to be two places at one time. Mom and Dad know. They see our love and loyalties multiply and divide and would do anything to help lighten our worries.

If only, I can't help but think sometimes as I stand in my backyard and wave to the elderly couple who live behind us while they tend to their garden or give their visiting grandkids rides on their very own golf cart.

If only, I often think as I look up and see those grandmas and grandpas with tan faces cheering boldly from the bleachers during my kids' basketball tournaments.

Hadn't my parents earned that sort of indulgence in their golden years, too?

Well . . . it is what it is. Not a pristine, round bouquet tied neatly in a bow. No, this life is never that. Rather, I like to think of it all as a gloriously sprawling cascade of rich, rustic wildflowers. Messy magnificence!

***

As I turn my attention back to the laptop screen, I hear Dad pulling into the garage. I click on the "File" menu and pull down to "Save." He's pretty good at remembering when I need to leave—I'm a wife and mother just as much as I'm a daughter.

My husband works until about seven o'clock tonight and has an hour commute. So, I'll pick up my son from the middle school for his orthodontist appointment. Then, I'll swing by the bus stop to pick up my younger daughter, because it's too cold for the walk home. Plus, I worry about her getting off the bus alone, strangers passing by, and . . . so many things. I'll run into the house to take out ground beef to thaw for dinner, although I have no idea what I'm going to make with it yet. Before the slew of evening activities begin, I'll pick up my older daughter from basketball practice at the high school—after grabbing a handful of chocolate chips and remembering where I set my car keys down. And, of course, I'll once again forget the overdue library books on the counter I'd planned to drop off on the way.

My children. They, too, pull me toward a love and longing impossible to define. There are no words to describe what I feel as I watch them standing at the free-throw line, curled up on the couch sleeping, or walking toward me while I wait for them in the car at the curb. Each of their life stories beginning, unfolding, adding freshness to a legacy of love bigger than themselves to which they'll forever belong—*just as God had willed them*, words from a mother's dream.

What's in store for them in years ahead when I'm no

longer able to pick them up or protect them? Will they one day know the poignancy of a life straddled and graced between two generations?

***

I'm no poet. Not like my mom. But if I were to wake up at an unseemly hour, not able to write down a dream poem that *must* come out, I have strong reason to believe my husband, a kind-hearted fella, would turn on the lamp, open the nightstand drawer, and pull out a piece of scratch paper and pen, too.

Maybe my poem would go something like this:

Life is squiggly, wiggly, wobbly,
doesn't follow our plan so snugly.
Its twists and turns sometimes the pits—
what's the object lesson in this?
Maybe it, too, is beyond describe
or found inside humbled beauty abound
who's doing her best with what she's able,
radiating from her lift chair near a messy old table.

By Julie Jo

Julie Jo Severson—co-curator and co-editor of this book—is a former PR girl now freelance writer, journalist, editor, and lost-and-found attendant of two teens and a tween. Still an English major at heart, she finds solace in writing her way through those universal experiences that bind us together. In 2015, she launched her storytelling blog Carvings on a Desk (www.carvingsonadesk.com) to reconnect with her own voice swirling around in the middle. Since then, her creative nonfiction has also been featured on Ten to Twenty Parenting, Midlife Boulevard, Mamalode, BonBon Break, and elsewhere. She lives in Minnesota with her husband of twenty-plus years and their three kids.

CHOOSING TO SAY YES
By Carol Heffernan

Last week, when my parents came for a visit, I was pretty sure my dad died while sitting on my leather couch. I noticed him drifting off during our conversation and at first didn't think much of it. At 92, he's lived well for decades with diabetes, but more recent diagnoses of cancer and Alzheimer's disease have taken a toll.

Still, he and my mom walk miles a day, unassisted, on wooded paths surrounding their senior housing. They try to beat their personal bests at Wii bowling (which my mom calls "Why bowling," confusing me for months!). In many ways, they have more robust social lives than I do.

In that moment, though, as I saw my dad's eyes closed, his mouth agape, his color slightly gray, I knew it was the end. I looked at him, my throat tightening, and here's what came to mind: *I thought I was ready for this. I'm not ready for this.*

As it turned out, I didn't have to be ready—not yet anyway—because shortly thereafter, my mom announced, "It's time to go," and my dad immediately replied, "Well, goodbye then," and smiled, eyes still closed.

A surprisingly lucid remark from someone who, most

days, doesn't recognize anyone around him. We've stood by as this thoroughly and hopelessly German man— opinionated, hardworking, stoic—has drifted further and further away from us. He smiles and greets everyone he sees in an effort to appear as if he knows you. But his vacant look gives him away. I remember the first time I saw "that look." I asked him a question at the dinner table, and my eyes widened as his lost focus. I don't think you forget moments like that. Thankfully, compared to other potential effects of this disease, my dad has only become more passive and gentle as the years have gone by.

Once, after he and my mom went to bed, he turned to her with a troubled expression and said, "Don't you think it's about time we start a family?"

My 83-year-old mother laughed and told him she thought seven kids and thirteen grandkids were plenty for now. He mulled that over for a bit and eventually agreed.

My dad grew up on a farm not far from where I live now but during a very different time in our country's history. A time when a big family, little money, lots of work, and no time for leisure were more commonplace. Farm life wasn't for him, so as soon as he could leave the country for the city, he did. He went to college, got a job in sales, and met my mom.

The two of them had a few things in common right from the start. My mom grew up on a farm. And she, too, came from a big family, little money, lots of work, and no time for leisure. Farm life wasn't for her, either, so as soon as she could leave the country for the city, she did. She went to college, got a job as a nurse, and met my dad.

Together, they bought a house in the suburbs and promptly filled it with six children. Nearly a decade after the birth of her sixth child, my mom started experiencing what she thought were early symptoms of menopause. As it turns out, she was pregnant at 44; my dad was 53.

And that's the story of how I wound up with parents whose AARP memberships arrived right around the time I started kindergarten. Like so many parts of childhood, I didn't know any different, so it never struck me as odd when I was asked why I lived with my grandparents.

I was in second grade when my dad retired, so I grew up with two parents at home. I had constant supervision, the latest large-print issues of *Reader's Digest*, a kitchen stocked with prune juice, oatmeal, and instant coffee, and no cable TV. ("Who needs all those channels?" my mom would ask with disgust). You know, just the typical stuff that makes a person really popular in high school.

Now, I have a 7-year-old daughter of my own, along with a 3-year-old son. It's interesting that my mom and I are both in the caretaker role, albeit for loved ones on opposite ends of a lifetime. When I take my toddler for our weekly visit to my parents, we like to explore together.

My mom holds my dad's hand, I hold my son's, and we walk carefully, slowly, carefully, slowly up and down the stairs and hallways.

We ask the one we're caring for the same questions, my mom and I: "Do you have to go to the bathroom?" "Did you sneak that last brownie from the counter?" "Are you sure you want to wear that coat when it's eighty degrees outside?" "Are your shoes on the right feet?" "Where did you hide my keys?" "Do you have to go to the bathroom?"

Sometimes, I'll call my mom in the early afternoon, and when I say, "My little guy is sleeping," she'll good-naturedly respond, "Mine is too."

Our two guys. They are different; they are the same.

I laughed last week when my dad arrived on our doorstep wearing worn jeans, a plaid shirt, and a straw fedora. As he and my mom stepped inside, my son burst into the room wearing worn jeans, a plaid shirt, and a straw fedora. I took a photo of the two sitting side by side on our porch swing, both squinting into the sunlight, eighty-nine years between them.

That was one of those ordinary, nothing-special days, really. But it's in those days that I see my parents' strength. Because, goodness knows, you need strength of steel to age gracefully. And, actually, you need it to parent gracefully, too.

To exhibit patience and good humor when you're asked the same question for the twentieth time. To make decision after decision, despite feeling ambivalent and just plain wrung out sometimes. To plan your day around someone else's delicate, well-worn routine.

That's what love is though, don't you think? Seeing the opportunity to put others before ourselves. And choosing, over and over again, to say, "Yes."

Carol Heffernan has written hundreds of articles about women's issues, health and wellness, and parenting. She is also a social media manager for a children's clothing company and interior designer. Carol lives in Wisconsin with her husband and two young (and very talkative just like their mother) children. She blogs at cpheffernan.wix. com.

DAD'S BOOKCASE
By Patricia Jonik Stein

My three sons and their father, "the guys," left for the ball game around eleven o'clock in the morning on Father's Day. This was a tradition they all enjoyed. It was a perfect day for a game—sunny, mild, and beautiful—and I was quite content staying home, cooking dinner, and working on a project I wanted to complete. It was also the first Father's Day we'd spend without my dad. I couldn't think of a more appropriate way to honor him than working on bookcases that had once belonged to his beloved brother.

My uncle had passed away a little before my dad died, and I had inherited some old barrister bookcases from an apartment he owned. They'd been nestled into a wall, and my cousin gladly removed them, but they were in need of much work before they would be once again usable.

Growing up, I spent many afternoons and evenings beside my dad on projects. He'd head down to the basement workshop in the house he and his brothers built and start tinkering or working on fixing something for my mother, my sister, or me. I'd often join him, sitting on the tall stool beside him while he showed me each step. He'd look around at the tools and array of usable items that littered his work bench until he found just the right thing to complete his task. Then he'd stand back and look over the project while he thought about the right way to proceed. He was the epitome of Rube Goldberg—that cartoonist and creator of fantastical, workable inventions—and could jury-rig anything and everything until, in some seemingly magical way, it worked.

Eventually, I married and established my own home, and Dad helped me upgrade and beautify my new surroundings. At my first house, he'd come after work and together we gutted, rearranged, and fixed the little starter house my husband and I purchased. He'd gather bits and pieces, odds and ends of wood, wire and tile and somehow work them into wonderful things. There was a much needed linen closet incorporated into an open second floor landing space, and a beautiful enclosed set of shelving replaced the broken broom closet in the dining room. With his expertise and my design, our little house became the showcase for the neighborhood. In due course, my family blossomed and outgrew the cozy cottage, and we found a new place to call home.

Dad, now retired, came and worked once again. I was the designer, and he turned my ideas into shelves, walls, cabinets, and a host of other household improvements. He added bannisters, fixed doors, and even mimicked the beautiful dining room shelves that were the centerpieces of my previous home. We worked together: I handed him tools and screws, and he hammered and measured while I designed the trim that would finish any given project. It was our way of being together, and our way of saying, "I love you," not with words, but with work.

I started on the top of the bookcases, having already cleaned and polished the wood. The tops had been split apart and needed to be put together and bolstered up to lay flat. I looked them over and tried to decide how Dad would fix them. Nails wouldn't hold, and there was no place to put screws. Then I remembered what my father often said, "Do what is simplest first, then if that doesn't work, try something else." With his words echoing through my mind, I decided that glue would do just fine, and I was right. While the glue set, I meandered into the kitchen and began cooking dinner, knowing the hungry guys would be returning soon.

I prepared a meal that had been a favorite of my dad, and also my husband; the same one I cooked every Father's Day. As I chopped and diced, I could almost feel my father smiling at me. I just knew he'd be proud of his daughter and her work. Once dinner was in the oven, it was time to get back to the bookcases.

The glue had set and the tops would now lay flat. There was a bit more prep work to do and as I set to work, I remembered those bygone days with my dad. He'd look at my designs and, in his words, "mull them over," then he'd shoot me a knowing glance, and we'd get to it.

He'd measure and cut, and then he'd drill holes to fit in the screws, which he preferred to nails, because they were easier to remove if the need should arise. As my mind drifted back through time, once again, I'd hand him tools and help measure, then help with the finishing touches; I returned to being his apprentice. But now, I needed to be the master.

As my reveries faded, it was time to leverage the tops onto the bookcases. I picked up the long, glued piece of wood and lifted it to crown the top of my uncle's bookcase. My five-foot, one-inch frame was no match for the top, and it tumbled onto the mechanism that held and worked the glass encased shelves. The metal broke, but luckily it missed the glass.

I looked at the metal, I looked at the glaring hole under the place where the top would rest, and I knew I had no idea how to fix it. I felt the tears start to well in my eyes, but stoically, like my dad would've wanted, I pulled apart the bookcase and examined the metal workings to see if there was a remedy. I tried, first the simplest method, then a more difficult one, to no avail. I simply didn't know what to do.

I'd worked so hard on the bookcase, and I'd so wanted it to look the way it had one hundred and fifty years ago when it was made. I wanted to make my dad proud of me. I thought about it, I turned it about in my head, and I tried to think like Dad had taught me. I failed.

There was clearly nothing I could do other than wish my father, with his magical hands, were there to fix it, as he had so many other things for me before. My mind rushed with the memories of my broken China mirror, a severed axle on a doll coach, a broken treasure box, and a small wounded record player—all put together by this wonderful, talented man, now gone almost a year.

I didn't want to give up, but dinner was done and my boys would be home soon. I felt defeated. As I retreated downstairs to finish dinner, I heard the front door slam with a resounding sound I was familiar with as my family returned from the game. I looked at my husband and sons, and the swells from my eyes burst open and streamed down my cheeks. I was disappointed in myself and frustrated, but most of all, I missed my dad terribly.

"What's wrong?" my sons asked almost in unison. As I told them, Christopher, my now adult middle child, asked me to show him. We went to the upper landing to the room that once had been his, and I showed him all the beautiful, ruined work I'd done on the bookcase.

He took the broken metal mechanism in his hands and turned it about. Suddenly, his blue eyes flashed that same knowing look I'd seen for so many years as I worked hand in hand with my dad.

"I can fix this. Pop taught me," he said with the same inflection I knew so well from my childhood. As this young man, my son, fixed my treasure and put it together, I knew my dad's legacy would live on and on through generations to come. I also knew Dad was not really far away, and that he'd always, in some way, be a part of my children and me.

Patricia Jonik Stein lives with her husband and two cats and writes from her Fort Washington, Pennsylvania home. She worked as a theme reader, writing coach, teacher, and mentor after a career in marketing research. She retired to care for her aging mother after her father's death. She raised three sons, who are now on their own, and she's happily awaiting the next generation to come along.

MY STRUGGLE WITH THE SUN
By Whitney Fleming

At the top of each hour, my mother climbs the stairs to administer drops in my eye. I'm sensitive to light, so I remain in the solitary confinement of my bedroom with its cloaked windows, a homemade cocoon blocking the outside elements. The sun is my kryptonite. My corneal nerves are enlarged due to a condition named acanthamoeba keratitis, which is short for parasites embedded in my left eye.

Sometimes between doses of the eye drops, she brings pain medication, a bottle of water, or a snack to encourage me to eat. Up and down the stairs she travels despite the painful arthritis in her hips.

"Vitamin C is a healer," she cajoles. "The nurses told me that after I had you, and it worked."

"Just have a little," my mother pleads, presenting me with a tray holding a bowl of crackers and a glass of orange juice, almost like an offering to the gods.

I shake my head and hold up my arm. "I can't. Not now."

"You have to eat," she states sternly, reminding me of nights at our family dinner table when I used to hide peas in my apple sauce.

"Thanks, but no," I whisper. "Maybe later."

Often, she holds my hand as I cry through the pain, stroking my hair like she did when I was young and suffered from the stomach flu or an earache. I sense her peeking through the crack of my bedroom door, and although I do not stir, the idea that she is checking on me warms my heart. Her presence is reassuring, as only a mother's is.

I hear her in the early morning, downstairs packing lunches, unloading the dishwasher, and clucking orders at my daughters to brush their hair and put folders in their backpacks. Laughter rings through the hallways and then a soft hushing reminder: "Not too loud, because I don't think your mom had a good night."

In the afternoons and evenings, she is busy fixing snacks and dinners, checking homework, and ensuring my daughters are on time for whatever carpool is arriving to shuttle them to and from their various activities.

Some days, when my husband is traveling or cannot leave work, she chauffeurs me to doctors' appointments. She never found her confidence behind the wheel, and I know she's flexing all her courage to drive in unfamiliar territory. As I meekly mumble directions with my eyes shielded beneath two pairs of sunglasses, she nervously chatters, telling me details about my children whom I barely spend time with the past few months.

When we arrive, she rushes around the car to the passenger side and takes my arm to lead me across the pavement and through automatic doors. It's with great irony I watch an elderly couple with canes step to the side to let us pass through first. What a sight we must be together, the mother and her sick daughter, yet at 42 years old, I'm hardly a child and she has added grandmother and great-grandmother to her role as mother.

As we wait, she reads a book or starts a grocery list. She checks my phone to confirm a text about a school project for one of my girls. She pats my leg and asks if I need anything.

It's a strange sensation to know the three-ringed circus of my household is operating as usual, yet without its ringleader. The day after her seventy-third birthday, my mother flew three-hundred miles to step in as my surrogate after I contracted a rare and debilitating eye disease that leaves me bed-ridden and visually impaired. While my husband is at work, she commandeers the ship while also caring for me.

It's a hefty burden for a woman who's in the sunset of her life. Surely she's done enough to earn a respite from the role of constant caretaker. The oldest of eight, she learned to change a diaper just after she was out of her own. Married at 18 and a mother a year later, she raised three kids staggered twelve years apart, and often offered refuge to family members who hit rough patches. When my father received his terminal lung cancer diagnosis after a five-decade smoking binge, she tirelessly tended to his every need and allowed him to die in his home with her arms lovingly wrapped around his frail body.

Her duty is done. It's her time to rest, her sunset to enjoy; yet, here she is, playing the role of caretaker again, mothering us all.

***

"It's just an exploratory test, a quick procedure. I'll be in and out the same day. The doctor doesn't think it's too serious, but they need to be sure. He wants me to go in soon, though." I hear my mother's words but find it difficult to process the information.

The sun is in my eyes as I try to focus on the road ahead, but the sound of my heart beating in my ears distracts me. I'm only a half mile from my driveway, but I pull my minivan over to the side of the tree-lined street to finish our phone call.

"I didn't even want to say anything as I don't want you to get upset," my mother states matter-of-factly.

"I can come, Mom. I can figure it out," I stutter. I begin mentally mapping out how I could manage to travel to Ohio, which, at the moment, feels like a trip to the moon. I put her on speakerphone and scan my calendar to see if my husband travels this week and what activities my three young daughters have on their schedules. My calendar is a sea of blue blocks of appointments, responsibilities, and obligations.

An internal tug o' war begins in my conscious. Just a year ago, my mother gave up her life to step into mine. It's time to return the favor, time to repay the debt, although I feel crushed by the weight of my obligations.

After months of begging her to visit a doctor for a urinary condition, I now want to take the pleading back. I stare at my white knuckles grasping the steering wheel as a thousand what-if scenarios swirl in my head. Cancer. Kidney failure. Blood disease. How could this happen to her after all she has done for everyone else?

"Nonsense," she barks. "You have too much going on, and who will watch the girls? Mark can't take any more time off after your being sick last year, and you're just getting back on your feet."

It's typical for my mother to be pragmatic in her time of need. It's her way. She's the caregiver, not the one to be cared for in any circumstance.

I'm frozen at the intersection of guilt and gratitude. I have a debt to repay, yet the lender won't call in her chit.

"Don't think about it again. I'll be fine. Now, I have to run, dear," she hastily remarks. "I'll talk to you later. Hugs to the girls!"

I don't get the chance to say my goodbye before she

hangs up the phone. I sit in my idling car for a few minutes, watching the world pass by with the fear that a piece of it may be ending. I contemplate a variety of scenarios so I can "be there" for my mother, my caretaker for the past forty-plus years, yet each one seems impossible at the moment.

***

A few weeks later, the sound of an old rotary phone ringing blasts loudly through my iPhone, signaling my mother is calling. As usual, I'm in the car, jetting home to make dinner after dropping my children off at activities. The days are getting slightly longer, and the setting sun is playing peek-a-boo through trees bursting with fresh leaves.

I take a deep breath as I pull off to the side of the road.

I barely spit out a "hello" before my mother says, "Everything is okay. They're going to monitor me, but all the tests came back negative."

I let out a squeal and my heart skips a beat. I hear the shakiness in her voice and the relief in her words. She was scared.

"I'm glad that's over," she tells me, going into detail regarding the procedure she endured.

She laughingly shares an interaction with a nurse who advised her to wash before sexual intercourse. "I kept telling her, lady, that ship has sailed, but she wouldn't let up." I almost feel the warmth of her smile through the phone.

I try to listen, but I can't control the rush of emotions surging through my brain like a tsunami.

I should've held her hand and brought her water. I should've whispered encouraging words. I should've walked her through the automatic doors of the doctor's office.

It's the way things should be in the mother-daughter relationship, yet it did not play out that way for us. Our roles were reversed to this point, and I'm keenly aware of it.

The guilt weighs heavy like a laden vest.

My mother and I are at an intersection of our relationship. She remembers what it's like to be busy with kids, a husband, a job, and the responsibilities that come with all of that.

None of that matters, however. She's not the only caretaker, the only curator of our tangled lives. I can—I will—help her in these sunset years.

"Mom," I interrupt. "I'm so glad you're okay, but next time something like this happens, I'm coming out to be with you. Or you can come here. It's my turn."

I hear her take a quick breath in to admonish me, but then a sigh emerges through the phone.

"Okay, dear. If that's what you want."

I hang up and feel relieved, almost empowered. I don't doubt my mother will be there for me as long as she has breath in her body, yet at last, she understands the feeling is reciprocated.

I put the car in drive and smile as I pull away from the curb. The last bits of light are dwindling as the sky turns a magnificent shade of purple. I hope my mom is looking out her window at this exact moment.

Sunsets are best when shared.

Whitney Fleming is a marketing consultant and freelance writer living outside Chicago. As the mother to three tween girls, she tries to dispel the myth that she is a typical suburban mom despite that she often is seen driving her minivan to PTA meetings and soccer practices. She blogs about parenting, relationships, and w(h)ine on Playdates on Fridays (www.playdatesonfridays.com), and regularly appears on sites such as Huffington Post (#Bestof2015), Scary Mommy, Mamalode, and Feminine Collective, among others. She recently appeared on the Animal Planet show "Monsters Inside Me" to discuss her experience with acanthamoeba keratitis, a debilitating eye condition caused by microscopic, water-born ameba.

LIVING, EVEN IN THE DYING
By Tina Porter

God, is it gorgeous today in Southern California. Nearly enough to make me fall in love with my hometown again. The hills are green, mountains a color that could almost be called purple (and, best of all, no smog so I can actually see them), and the sky is brilliant blue. There are oranges on the trees, pink and red flowers in bloom, and I'm sitting between two open doors with a breeze that carries me from one vista to another.

We're in that time, as a family, that's out of time. I suppose you could read that either way: living beyond time or living with little left. Both are true.

I'm typing this as a man sets up a hospital bed in my parents' family room. My father will be brought home in a few hours, officially on hospice. One sister is on her way from South Carolina; another sister will be arriving from Arizona tomorrow; and our brother will be back in town on Saturday, the day I'm scheduled to go back home to Indiana.

But what kind of schedule can we be on now?

I've been here since Saturday; my father's been in the hospital since Friday. They've been working so hard at making him, with stage four lymphoma, stronger, and I can't help but ask, for what?

I went to the hospital this morning to have breakfast with him while my mother took care of some business at home. He laid in that big old bed that only looked big because of the stark smallness the cancer brought with it. He wore a dark blue cap on his hairless head, his ears sticking out from underneath it, and he was just so happy to have woken up one more day (though he didn't say so).

***

It's a new day, and my dad is home laying in that bed the man set up, trying not to fall asleep. His good friend, Bob, is supposed to be coming over, and he wants to be awake to visit with him.

I'm grateful, right now. Seems like a silly time to be so, but I'm here, with my folks, my siblings here, too, or soon arriving, and my father awake, knowing what's coming—all of us knowing what's coming. This is an easy place to be, the place without denial, the place of acceptance. The place of just being.

I should be more anxious. Truthfully, it was more stressful before, when I was back in Indiana trying to decide when to come here to California again to be with my parents. Two months ago, I brought my husband and kids here for a week-long vacation during which I tried to gauge the situation, already certain there'd be no more holidays with my dad. Then we returned to Indiana, and

I buried my head in the sand of daily duties that revolve around a family of five with two working parents. I 'angsted' (as my mother says) about it relentlessly— should I go back? How about now? Now? Maybe now?

And then my mom called to say he was in the emergency room, that he'd woken up with chest pains, this survivor of two heart attacks, and that she'd called the paramedics, forgetting, for the moment, that he had lung cancer. She called me again late in the evening, and I could hear the strain in her voice as she told me that after twelve hours, he was still waiting to be admitted, to get off the gurney in the hall, and I didn't equivocate any longer.

By the time I arrived at the hospital, Dad was getting food through IVs and having hallucinations brought on by dehydration. On Sunday, he was lucid again, enough so the doctor presented him with two choices: he could be released to a rehabilitation center to continue to get stronger so he could resume his chemotherapy, or, he could go home with only a palliative care regime. Hospice.

Hospice—the word I'd been waiting for someone to say, and I held my breath, waiting for my father's response. It was obvious from the moment I arrived on Saturday, we were nearing the end. But by Sunday, full of nutrients he'd not been getting enough of at home, because eating was just too hard, he had the sparkle in his eyes and even jumped out of bed to walk the length of his room (with a walker) at least twice. Then, the doctor gave him those two choices, and his demeanor changed profoundly.

"I want to go home," he said quietly, to my mom, while I gave up the pretense of not eavesdropping from the other side of the drape.

And so he did.

We laugh, here. We laugh about life, about plans, about whether we should do this or that and when. As we live "out of time," there seems to be no reason to worry about any of it. At all.

Of course, it's easy right now, because he's sitting up and talking and eating ice cream. And we have all slept as much as we could. And my mother is thrilled to have this time with him, eating ice cream at ten-thirty in the morning because, and for no other reason, she can.

***

The week is now over for me. Tomorrow I get on a plane back home to my kids, my cats, my husband, and the snow—most of which I'm thrilled about. And yet, I leave my hometown, and in doing so, must say goodbye to my father.

My father taught Communications for many years at a community college; throughout his tenure, student facilitators helped him teach. A few months ago, those facilitators gathered together for a reunion here at my parents' house. One of them called the other day while my mother was otherwise occupied, and I took the call. "He's my hero," she said of my dad, "and she's my other hero," she said of my mom.

"Mine, too," I said.

Today, that's never been more true—despite teenage years shouting just the opposite. This is hard stuff they're going through, but they make it easier for themselves and for us by facing it straight on. My father has not balked about any of the work we've done these last few days to keep him clean and comfortable. Nor has he complained about where his bed is or griped at all about being handed about like a stiff, unwieldy doll.

More though, is Mother my hero today. She extends her love through advocating for the best care, now that she can control it, now that his life is almost over. She kisses him good morning and goodnight and several times throughout the day. She cares for him, she cares about him, and she does it all with humor and aplomb. She pays attention to what matters in these waning days and dismisses the rest.

She breathes in and breathes out and faces what's next with both feet planted firmly on the ground. She doesn't like it but accepts it. Her heart is breaking. But she keeps on, because this is living, even in the dying.

She is superhuman, this mother of mine. My father is, too, were that he immortal.

My mother and sisters and I confer, agreeing that I need to head home, that I need to tend to my other family, the children and husband I left behind, who fend without me, supporting me unseen. I leave, then, and will not stay these last days of my father's life. This week has been enough, I tell myself. It has to have been enough. I'm honored to have been given the opportunity to serve him, to care for him, to make him grilled cheese sandwiches, to change his bedclothes, to be one of those he looks to with wide eyes, willing himself, it seems, to see fully, maybe for the first time ever.

I leave my heroes in the capable hands of my siblings, and though I'm angry at the medical system for making my father wait in the waiting room for so long, I'm also strangely grateful. The emergency situation required me to make a decision to come sooner than I'd planned, and with an urgency I hadn't prepared myself for, regardless of the truths before me. It led me here, to be of service, and to witness and experience this excruciatingly beautiful time in my parents' lives, in my life.

This is what we are here for, is it not? To be of use, to love, to neither dodge nor deflect the difficult, to understand the difference between what sort of matters and what ultimately and always matters.

There is no goodbye that can adequately cover this—except the goodbye that embraces the life I live, the

goodbye that deepens the human experience, the goodbye
that turns experiences back out.

***

A week later, I'm sitting in the auditorium of the
middle school for my daughter's band performance. I
have my cell phone in hand, which is not normal practice
for me, and I keep looking at it, until I realize, there's
no cell phone reception. I'm panic-struck at not being
available to my California family while also realizing
I'm not any more available to my Indiana family, missing
everything right in front of me. This is the game now, I
think. "Between and betwixt," my mother always used to
say. I'm neither fully one place nor another.

Dad died shortly after the concert. When we flew home
after the funeral, my husband, who needs back surgery,
walked with a cane that had belonged to my grandmother
and that had been at my parents' house. His back was
so bad, there was no relief either in sitting, standing, or
sleeping. As I sat in the airport, watching people maneuver
around him gingerly, I wondered why no one was doing
the same for me. Weren't my wounds visible enough, a
loss so great, even in the inevitability of it?

Once home, I tried to remember to pay the bills and
feed the kids and empty the dishwasher. I pretended to be
the mom they'd come to rely on. Eventually, about the
time my eldest grabbed my attention by saying I wasn't

paying any attention to her, I came back, inch by inch.

There's no way out but through, and through I go, by way of attending to whomever is present, right now, and with my feet planted firmly on the ground. Just like my parents modeled for me.

Tina Porter is a writer living in Northwest Indiana. She and her husband recently celebrated twenty-five years of marriage and the college graduation of their first born. Her middle and youngest daughters continue their sister's legacy at Indiana University, Bloomington. Her mother continues to be her hero. Tina was selected as an artist in the Valparaiso Community Supported Arts program for her poetry. You can read more of her work at tinalbporter. com.

A BROTHER THING
By Melissa Janisin

Sometime in the late 1980s, somewhere along the shoulder of Route 376 East in Pittsburgh, four people stand around a wrecked car. I'm one of them. My friend Heather, my dad, and his brother Albert are the others. We've just been to a Pittsburgh Pirates game. None of us are hurt, the car is entirely drivable, but Heather and I, aged 16 or so, have concert tickets for later and are anxious to be on our way. The police have come and logged their report. It seems we are about to be set free. Until:

Police Officer: So, you're sure you're all right? No injuries? No pain?

Dad: Huh . . . now that you mention it. Does my neck hurt? (*He feels his neck with his hand, as if this makes any sense whatsoever*)

Uncle Albert: Who are you asking, Ej? We don't know about your neck. Does it hurt, or what?

Dad: (*Twisting his head all around quite freely*) I don't know! It might hurt. Or, what if it hurts later? I can't tell.

Me: DAD! It either hurts, or it doesn't.

Dad: Well, then it does, I guess. Wait, does it?

Me: (*In my teenagery voice*) OH MY GOD!

Heather: (*Remains polite*)

Uncle Albert: Ej, you're the only person I know who can't tell if his own damn neck hurts him or not.

Dad: (*Chuckles*)

Me: (*Gritting my teeth*) IT'S NOT FUNNY—WE HAVE A CONCERT TO GO TO AND WE NEED TO GET HOME.

Dad: (*To police officer*) Well, can I call you later if I decide it hurts?

Police Officer: Me, personally?

And so on.

The remarkable thing about this day to me, other than Heather's and my rather extreme lack of concern for anything except our future musical entertainment, is that it perfectly represented a typical scene between my dad and his brother. Dad was the uncertain, impressionable, little brother; Uncle Albert was the one who told him how things needed to be. Not that my dad ever seemed to mind. "Sure, Al," he'd say, upon being told to "put the saw down already and let me do it."

"Albert says we need to," he'd tell my mother, taking a sledgehammer to the tile in their bathroom.

"My deepest sympathy," he said to Uncle Albert, when their brother Ben passed away.

"Ej," said Uncle Albert. "He was your brother, too."

As for me, I always liked being around the two of them,

primarily because I almost never had to talk if I didn't want to. Which is not to say that we enjoyed frequent stretches of companionable silence. On the contrary, what I mean is that in the company of my dad and Uncle Albert, all speaking parts were accounted for. This was how they got along—noise.

I mostly knew this thanks to the seven thousand or so Pirates games I'd attended with them, prior to the day of The Car Wreck. Pirate games were a big thing for us, the two of them cursing through nine innings while I sat between them, reading and re-reading my program.

"What the hell, Ej, look at that guy. He's pretty damn short for a first baseman."

"Who, him? He's taller than me, what do you mean?"

"I hope he's taller than you! What are you, five foot two? Three? Mis, how tall is your dad, huh?"

"I don't—"

"I'm five foot eight."

"And still too damn short to play first base. Am I right, Mis?"

And so on.

Of course, that was all a long time ago. Uncle Al is now 84, my dad is nearly 80. Uncle Al is easily as healthy as me. My dad is, too, aside from the Alzheimer's disease. One true fact about Alzheimer's—it changes the dynamic.

And now here we were, Uncle Albert and I, going to

visit my dad/his little brother at the nursing home. On the way there, he asks me, "Do you think this place is good for him, Mis?" And I have told him, "I don't know." Because I don't. Does anyone ever?

The good news is that my dad is awake when we get there, or at least, sitting upright in the TV room and not laying in his bed. "Oh, hey," he says, when he sees his brother and me. "What are you doing here?"

"We came to see you," says Uncle Albert. "How are they treating you, huh? How do you like this place?"

"Yeah . . . it's good," says my dad. "Good. I was just . . . you know. I don't know what I was doing."

Here, with another visitor, a moment of awkward silence might ensue; not so with Uncle Al. He's happy to jump right into the realm of the impossible Alzheimer's conversation. God love him.

"You look good, Ej," he says now, very kindly, because the truth is my dad is kind of a mess on this particular day. His hair is way too long, his glasses are lost, and he hasn't shaved in days. Plus, he's missing two teeth, which has been true for quite a while but still doesn't do much to improve the overall effect.

"Yeah, thanks," says my dad, adjusting the baseball cap which he rarely takes off. "I was just, you know. Sitting here."

Uncle Al looks pained, but keeps going, keeps talking

and engaging my dad in a way I never do. I don't think I can. It's just something between them, I guess, and it's clear to me that though he may be somewhat nervous and almost entirely clueless, my dad is happy to be the object of someone's attention. To be a central part of a conversation, even if he has no idea how it's supposed to go. To be talking with his brother.

My own kids, brothers at the current ages of 7 and 8, are friends only at my most optimistic moments. They get along, about half the time. They also fight, argue, brawl, and use the term "arch nemesis" correctly, in reference to each other. I desperately hope they will grow up to be real friends, drinking buddies, each the other's best man. I hope they will take their children to Pirates games together. I rarely consider the "nursing home pals" scenario.

"Yeah, you remember that, Ej?" says Uncle Albert now. "You remember playing the trumpet?"

"Trumpet?" says my dad and then stares into the distance for a moment. Or more.

"You were good," Uncle Al tells him. "You were in a band."

"Yeah," says my dad, vaguely. Then, "Your hair"—he points at his brother's head—"It looks nice. You got a lot of hair. More than me, haha."

He's been saying this forever. It's kind of amazing, the random things he holds on to. And I know a time will come when he'll no longer say it, when he'll forgot his brother altogether, but for now, it's still there. Whatever it is. Maybe it's a brother thing. I hope it's a brother thing.

I can't imagine, nor do I have any reason to imagine, my own kids at these advanced ages.

Still, I really, really hope it's a brother thing.

Melissa Janisin is a mom of two and stepmom of one, living and working in Pittsburgh, Pennsylvania. She writes about her life as a mom, wife, and daughter at www.goodnessmadness.com.

THE MUSIC STAND
By Lisa Pawlak

As far back as I can remember into my childhood, my mom, an evening and weekend flutist, would dress in elegant black "pit" clothing, collect her various musical wares—flute, piccolo, sheet music, and collapsible music stand—and head off to whatever show she was currently playing in.

She had quite a few instruments, including several flutes, one of which was her standard, but there was also the hole-less key one, and the one that had belonged to my grandfather, who'd been a professional musician. She also had a piccolo, oboe, and clarinet. I believe most of her instruments were passed on to my musical younger brother, appropriately so, when Mom died just over thirteen years ago. I'd guess the instruments are worth a fair amount of money.

Unlike the instruments, the music stand she'd tote along on those many nights and weekends was nothing of any monetary value. I saw something similar recently for fifteen dollars. But as a child, I used to love to put it together for her. It was in two pieces: the bottom base opened up like a tripod, with the top part attaching to it and folding down from the middle like a fan, to embrace her sheet music. It was shiny silver and you had to be careful with it—parts of it were pokey, and sometimes I'd get a little scrape. Thoughts of Mom's music stand still fill me with the warmth of her practicing, with images of her dressed all in black and, for some reason, with the sound of her laughter.

My son, Joshua, took up his first musical instrument, the ukulele, at the age of 7. Each time he practiced, he'd build a makeshift music stand out of various couch pillows, against which he'd lean his music binder and sit cross-legged in front to play. Impromptu music stand or not, I could see that Joshua was already showing much promise as a musician.

Soon after Joshua took up the ukulele, my dad planned a trip to visit us—my husband, my two boys, and me—and asked what type of gifts he could bring along for the boys. I don't remember what I suggested for Jonah, probably a Star Wars action figure or something like that, but for Joshua, I immediately suggested a music stand. "Nothing ornate or expensive," I clarified, since I was, of course, thinking of one like Mom's.

Dad surprised me when he told me he still had Mom's music stand and would be happy to bring it for Joshua. That was wonderful—not only did I know Joshua would love it, I also knew Mom would've loved for Joshua to have it. She may have initially laughed at the idea of all the attached sentimentality, because I could've just gone out and bought one.

Her true pride-and-joy music stand was still back at Dad's house—mahogany? Or was it teak? It was now tilted farther back than it used to be with the giant Webster's dictionary, one of Dad's pride-and-joys, displayed open on top. But she didn't get that one until later, probably after I'd gone off to college.

Dad asked me if it was okay for Joshua to get a used one; he could get a new one for him if it mattered, and I, of course, assured him this particular used one was just fine.

In addition to the music stand, Dad would also be bringing Gloria, his new girlfriend, with him. Since Mom died, Dad has had several girlfriends, but Gloria was the first, and only, one he brought to visit us. I hadn't met her before. Throughout the visit, I was relieved to find Gloria kind and fun to be around. And while parts of the week were a little rough to stomach—it was early in their relationship, if you can imagine some of the awkward moments—overall, I was happy that Dad had met someone.

Just before they traveled, Dad mentioned on the phone he had the music stand packed and would be sure to make a big deal to Joshua that it had belonged to his Grandma Gail. I was touched that Dad also seemed to attach sentimentality to this particular music stand, although in retrospect, I suppose I should've already figured that out by the mere fact he'd kept it for years. But he had no need for such an object anymore.

One evening during Dad and Gloria's visit, while the "grown-ups" sat around drinking mai-tais, Joshua announced he'd be giving a concert playing his ukulele. Dad looked at me and said, "This sounds like a good moment for the gift."

I smiled and went into the kitchen to deal with dinner and let them have their moment, while listening into the other room for Joshua's reaction. And his reaction was predictably pleasurable; he squealed with delight, immediately set it up, and ran to his room to retrieve his ukulele and music sheets for the concert.

Meanwhile, in the next room, I sighed, feeling as if the whole world had just shifted.

As Dad presented the gift to Joshua—the music stand I'd so adored as a child, the music stand he'd held on to for the past five years until the exact right moment he could part with it, the music stand he'd assured me Joshua would know was his Grandma Gail's—the only words he spoke were, "This is a gift from Gloria and me."

At some point during the visit, and it must've been before the shocking presentation, Dad told me he'd taken a razor blade and painstakingly scraped off a well-adhered piece of masking tape from the music stand, on which my mom had written her name. He seemed quite pleased with himself for making such efforts. But, I wished he hadn't done that. He'd made such an effort to remove what so surely belonged.

My initial reaction related to the thought of no longer seeing Mom's writing, which had been perfect and beautiful; the memory of which made me ache inside. I wanted to see that piece of tape, to envision her carefully writing her name on it and attaching it to the music stand where it would stay for years to come.

What leaves a more lasting impression, however, is how out of proportion that act of removal was, the very deliberate amount of time and effort Dad put into scraping off Mom's name versus the absolute lack of thought and sensitivity he put into its relabeling when he declared it to be from "Gloria and me." Everything he should've said was left silent.

I should've said something right then, right at that moment, right when it happened. I should've said something, *anything*, that very night.

I should've pointed out that even though he'd scraped off her name, even though he'd said it was a gift from "Gloria and me," it was *Mom's* music stand and it was being passed down to Joshua, her first grandchild. This music stand would give him a connection to the grandmother whom he couldn't remember but who had loved him every bit as much as I do. When I think about all this now, I like to think I said nothing simply because I was in shock by Dad's proclamation, and there is probably a certain amount of truth to that.

What feels closer to the mark, though, is that I said nothing because I lacked the courage to do so. I lacked the courage to invite my mom back into that room with us, to force my dad to acknowledge her presence, to reintroduce her into our conversations, and to reawaken memories of her music, her laughter, and her loss.

Years have passed, and, still, my mom's name is rarely mentioned in my dad's presence. In all of these years, it still upsets me that I didn't say anything to my dad about the presentation of the music stand. At times, I feel his actions that day, and my lack thereof, ultimately affected our entire relationship.

I sometimes wonder if it's not too late to find the courage to rewrite my mom's name. Perhaps, together, we could use indelible ink and carefully place her name back into our lives, where it belongs.

Lisa Pawlak is a San Diego-based freelance writer and regular contributor to the Chicken Soup for the Soul *series,* San Diego Family, Carlsbad *and* Hawaii Parent *magazines. Her work can also be found in Scary Mommy-Club Mid,* Coping with Cancer Magazine, *the* Christian Science Monitor, *Mothers Always Write, Sweatpants & Coffee, Mamalode, Imperfect Parent, and* Working Mother Magazine. *Lisa is also expecting publication in several upcoming anthologies.*

A PRAYER FOR SERENITY
By Jeanine DeHoney

"God, give me grace to accept with serenity
the things that cannot be changed,
courage to change the things
which should be changed,
and the wisdom to distinguish
the one from the other."
—The Serenity Prayer

I hear my mother's voice on nights when slumber evades me. "I'm going home tomorrow, right?" she shouts like a child in the midst of a temper tantrum.

"You can go home as soon as you get better," I tell her as I stroke her silver hair.

Her eyes search for the truth. She knows I'm lying.

Although I'd prayed for her miraculous recovery from heart disease, her prognosis was grim. My mother's insurance only allowed her to have a home attendant for four hours each day. So my older sister and I and my aunt took turns caring for her after we left work, in the apartment she lived in for over forty years and raised us kids in. Even though the area had changed not for the best and her good friends who'd lived above and below her had long moved away, she swore she'd never leave this place that was full of her sweetest memories—not willingly anyway.

I was always on edge wondering how I'd care for her as she got progressively worse. I'd rush to take over for either the health-aide worker, my aunt, or my sister but would sometimes feel so drained from my own day of working as a preschool teacher, I'd be on the verge of tears when I saw her. Reality sat on my shoulders like a ton of bricks as I grasped she'd never be well again. It was hard to handle without breaking down.

I tried my best to do the physical things and other tasks to care for her. I kept a diary of what she ate, doled out her medications, fixed her special meals, sponge bathed her, but I had difficulty lifting her off her hospital bed to use the bathroom, which she insisted on using. I tried to appease her, shunning the visiting nurse's voice about her using the bedpan so she wouldn't fall, knowing that using the bathroom was my mom's way of holding on to her dignity.

And when she slept, I watched her closely, my phone always in my hand to call the ambulance each time she motioned she couldn't breathe, which seemed to happen once a week. Whenever the paramedics came, my own heart weakened. I wasn't ready to be motherless.

Often as I turned the key in my mother's fifth floor

apartment, I took a deep breath and asked for serenity. And one day, when again I had to wait excruciating minutes for an ambulance to arrive, I made the most regretful decision I'd ever make with my sister: to put our mother in a nursing home.

It wasn't the place we wanted to see her in. She'd cared for my sister and me all of our lives until we left home. She deserved to be in the place where she'd carved familial memories. During the transition, I had a constant stomachache. When I went to the doctor, she told me it was most likely stress. I started crying in her office and told her about my mother. Deep down, I knew it was guilt pressing on my heart, my emotional organs.

God give me the grace I need to accept with serenity this decision we have made for our mother.

I cushioned my words when I talked to my mother. How could I tell her the home that gave my sister and me roots and wings would no longer be the place she could come back to? How could I tell her she had a new address and only a room now to call her own?

This wasn't a fairy tale or a dream I could wake up from. I couldn't click my heels as I held my mother's frail hand and take her back home like Dorothy and Toto. So I asked for serenity instead.

***

My sister and I found a place that a friend of my sister's

father was in. We scrutinized the facility and its staff with a fine-tooth comb and found it to be a comfortable haven for her and close enough for us to visit daily. Still, I was the one ranting and raving and having a temper tantrum. I didn't like this place my mother was in. Who were these people that thought it was fine to ask me to leave the room when they bathed her? I wanted to see whether they lifted the folds of her skin and washed the crevices of her body with warm enough water, as tenderly as I did when she was at home. They didn't know she liked to wear rose lipstick from Avon, and that even if she never wrote, she wanted a pen and pad of paper on her nightstand.

My mother wanted to sleep all day, but the attendants insisted she go to the day room to watch TV, but they never had on any of the shows she liked. No court shows, no documentaries on PBS. They played music but never the jazz my mother loved and that would've made her smile and remember my father who played the saxophone.

Sometimes they did arts and crafts with glitter, like I did with my preschoolers, to make Valentine's Day cards. I could see her face crinkle with a grimace thinking how juvenile this was. She would've preferred a set of watercolors and an easel to paint on if she could've mustered up enough strength to be artistic.

I felt nauseated. When would my serenity come?

At one point, I contemplated leaving my job to take

care of her after seeing her sadness. But even though my husband would've supported my decision, I didn't want to lay all of our own mounting financial responsibilities at his feet.

My mother was silent more than usual whenever I visited her. She stopped asking when she was going home, but I could see her eyes still questioning me. Soon she refused to eat or drink, and they had to feed her intravenously. She was giving up.

We hadn't told her that her belongings were packed away in boxes. She didn't know that soon a new tenant's belongings would fill the rooms that were once hers, ours. I couldn't bear to tell her. I said her goodbyes for her and lingered in those places I knew she would: her bedroom, the kitchen, her perch near the window.

***

My mother died four months after entering the nursing home. The last month of her life was spent in the intensive care unit of a nearby hospital. In some way, I feel she planned it this way. She wanted to be in a place where there was the miracle of birth, where broken limbs got mended, and where the majority of people recovered from their illnesses and went home.

It's taken me years to absolve myself of the guilt about our decision to put her in a nursing home. Although I wish I could've written a different beginning to this story, one in which I talked about caring for my mother in her home until her passing, I know if she could, she'd hold me in her arms and absolve me of all guilt. She'd remind me how I brushed her hair, sang to her, prayed out loud for her, and sat for hours holding her hand. Serenity eventually came, slowly like sand in an hourglass. I realized I didn't always have to be oak-tree strong. And in the midst of my journey, I was granted the wisdom to offer reassuring words to others walking in my worn shoes as a caretaker of aging parents, so they, too, can one day have serenity to carry them through.

Jeanine DeHoney is a former Family Services Coordinator and Art Enrichment Teacher. As a freelance writer, her work can be found in Timbuktu, Mused-Bella Online, Skipping Stones Multicultural Magazine, *online at This I Believe, The Write Place At The Write Time, Literary Mama, Underwater NYC, Mutha Magazine, The Mom Egg, True Stories Well Told, Devozine, Writing For Dollars, Empowerment for Women, My Brown Baby, Wow: Women on Writing—The Muffin's Friday Speak-out, Metro Fiction, Scary Mommy.com and Parent Co. and The Artist Unleashed. She is an essayist in* Chicken Soup for the African American Woman's Soul *and contributing writer to* Dream Teen Magazine. *She was also the 2014 winner of The Brooklyn Art and Film Festivals Nonfiction Contest.*

WE COOK
By Carol A. Cassara

In Memory of Marilyn

We cook.

When we don't know what else to do, we cook.

Seasoned tri-tip roast nestled in a bed of organic broccoli slow-cooked to palate-tempting perfection. Beef for stronger blood, broccoli to repair the immune system. Dishing out hope against hope, heaping spoonfuls of guarded promise carefully plated and set on the table.

Pulling a big knife from the block, I chop watermelon into sweet red cubes, dice redolent minty green leaves, and section an orange. Sprinkling feta cheese over the mix, I serve it up on a white plate, a life-restoring offering.

If only.

I stand over a stainless steel pot of black beans infused with onion, garlic, and spices, my wooden spoon moving in slow circles to meld the flavors, my nose twitching at the aromas. She loves my black beans and will ask for them several times this week. How little it is, but it is all I can do. We're all helpless when we see death in the waiting room, biding its time.

Broad layers of pasta noodles in the casserole topped with meat, yellow and green vegetables, and scarlet marinara remind me of the cooking course the two of us took outside of Rome that autumn week all those years ago. We cooked two huge meals a day—and ate them— laughing the whole time, learning from Italians who had no English. We were fluent in the language of the kitchen, and we speak it still, even as we watch the stopwatch tick steadily the minutes of her life, of our lives.

We will speak that language until the end.

How did we get here so fast? I wonder as carrots, zucchini, onion, and green beans simmer in the soup pot, my face hot in the steam, holding my tears in the corner of my eyes, blotting them before they fall. I'm afraid if I let them go they won't stop: tears for the women we once were and the women we are now, but mostly for what she's going through, her disease picking up speed now. The doctors can't infuse bags of blood and platelets fast enough to keep up with the disease. I can't infuse food fast enough either.

I didn't draw a lucky family card and longed for the kind of sister mine would never be. I was 33 when I found someone better—this sister-friend who is now dying.

Who can explain the alchemy of sisterhood, when masks drop away and souls connect? How is it that we can have it with one person and not another? What will I do when she's gone?

We've sat together at many tables, for meals, for

cocktails, pouring wine and pouring out our souls. Now, she insists on rolling her walker to the dinner table and sitting for as long as her disease will let her, even if it's just minutes.

Through onion tears, I can barely see the knife move on the cutting board. If I'm not careful I could slice my finger and I almost want to, to feel something other than gut-wrenching sorrow.

Endings have never been my strength; I've always kept people in my life long after the relationship wilted around the edges. But this one stayed fresh through each stage of our lives, though we had little in common—nothing obvious, anyway.

I grab seasonings from my spice rack. She's always loved her food spicy, but now it takes more than simple spices to tempt her palate. I double my usual measured spoonfuls and add oregano and seasoned pepper to the waiting stock pot, and finally, hot pepper.

When we met, she was a stay-at-home wife of a prosperous executive and mother of two. Divorced twice and childless, I was trying desperately to find a job in a new city, new state, and new industry. Her long, graceful fingers sparkled with diamonds and gold, while my one solitaire sat in a drawer, a symbol of my failed marriage. Her friends were all "ladies who lunched," and I was a woman with a briefcase and a 1980s business suit.

But we "got" each other instantly. Maybe it was because we shared Italian heritage, maybe because we were both transplanted Californians from the northeast. I can't explain it, and really, it's not important. What's important is that we connected. It stuck, too. Our bond carried us more than thirty years, through love affairs, divorces, and remarriage; through new jobs and graduations; through earthquakes, dinners in Italy, and wine drunk in Napa. And through secrets, both shared and unshared.

Later, our connection carried us through ambulance rides to the emergency room, three different wheelchairs, two walkers, and stints in the intensive care unit; through chemotherapy, opportunistic infections, and, then, through celebrations of miraculous rallies. Now, though, in a final test, it's carrying us through her death.

That thirty-year span of friendship was unfathomable when we met, but now, as the end is foreshadowed, I'm startled at how quickly the days have passed and are still speeding by, way too fast. I want to stop time, freeze it in place, keep her with me. I cannot fathom the world otherwise.

I hold on to the cutting board as if I were holding on to her life, chopping furiously, angry at the loss to come, each chop a *No!* half pleading and half demanding.

Broth is simmering on the stove, waiting for me to add the last cup of her favorite vegetables. She'll have the soup for dinner tonight, served hot, not lukewarm. She hates her food lukewarm.

I scoop bright green florets of broccolini into the water, add seasoning, and cook.

Carol A. Cassara is a writer whose essays have appeared in Skirt!, *the* Christian Science Monitor, Blood and Thunder *literary magazine, the* San Francisco Chronicle, Tampa Tribune, Syracuse Post-Standard, *on KQED public radio, on PBS' website, Next Avenue, in the anthology* Dumped: Women Unfriending Women, *in several* Chicken Soup for the Soul *books and other publications and anthologies. When she's not writing, she's traveling the world with her awesome husband or playing with her adorable, but bratty, maltipoo. Her blog, Heart-Mind-Soul inspires reader to create their best lives: www.carolcassara.com.*

GRANDPARENT PRIVILEGE
By Jackie Pick

"Do you think they'll be okay?"

I stretch out uncomfortably in the passenger seat, disrupting a jury-rigged garbage bag, two backpacks, and my purse which, at last count, had three Tide pens, a travel pack of tissues, and a bag of goldfish crackers.

In answer to my question, my husband tilts his head toward the back seat. One child has already tried to unbuckle his seatbelt, another is rolling the window down to "smell the Grandma air," which is, as he puts it, "fresher," and the youngest is leaning forward against her seatbelt as if to push the car on just a little faster. "I think they'll be fine," he says.

"I meant my parents."

We've long referred to my parents' house as Vegas. After a visit, the kids return buzzing from the open juice bar, carrying gift bags, and experiencing a vague disappointment that regular life doesn't involve a twenty-four-hour buffet and turndown service. The entertainment factor there is high, as are my children's expectations.

My kids have been planning for this overnight for weeks, making sure to do nothing that would jeopardize the event. They packed their bags without being asked (and actually packed what they needed), practiced table manners ("Grandma would want us to put our napkins on our laps!"), and went to bed without complaint. Anytime we dealt with a minor rule infraction, their eyes would grow big with worry. "I still get to go to Grandma's, right?" They were ready and eager, and that type of anticipation can only lead to a type of behavior best described as *volcanic*.

My parents, on the other hand, hadn't had to deal with three young children for more than a few hours at a time in decades. They were out of practice, their own routines calcified, their noise and chaos tolerance, never stellar, had to have decayed into a permanent state of rot by now. Although my parents had the homefield advantage, not to mention more experience and height, I had to give the edge to the kids. They brought to this event noise, conspiracy, and nearly immeasurable kinetic energy augmented by the promise of junk food and the absence of their mother reminding them how to behave every three seconds.

Surely, my parents were doomed to a week's recovery in a darkened room.

The car decelerates, and all the junk on the floor rolls forward; the bags in the back, packed to excess as though the kids were going on an expedition rather than just an overnight at Grandma's, lurch forward, bonking the children, who giggle at this sign of our final approach.

Were it not for the safety locks on the doors, they would've exited the car a block early. As it is, we barely turn the engine off before they shoulder-roll out the door.

***

My mother senses our advent and opens the front door before the kids get a chance to work the doorbell like quality control experts. My mother looks put-together. Her hair is styled, her outfit classic with modern touches, and she smells terrific. I absent-mindedly finger a hole in the thigh of my jogging pants.

She quickly turns her attention to the children. The check-in procedure is chaotic as the kids quickly make themselves comfortable. They throw their shoes off as they take off coats, laugh-scream their arrival, shake off dogs, and run for hugs in tactical formation. My mom jumps into the fray and lavishes them with kisses while helping them take off their coats. In return, after the affection supernova, they're "interrogated" about goings-on at school: Did they do well on their spelling tests? Which of their classmates has athlete's foot? Who has seen the newest juice box design? Their answers are excited and detailed.

Last night at dinner, I also asked them questions: "How was school? Who did you sit next to at lunch? What are you doing in math? What was the best thing that happened to you today?" The answer to each of these was

"Fine" or "Alex." They crammed food into their mouths so they could be excused quickly and run around like feral monkeys until their baths.

My father emerges with his hand-drawn map, labeled "Grandma's House" (it's never referred to as "Grandpa's House" for reasons unclear). Each room has been transformed into thematic stations: The family room is the Puzzle and Train Room, the kitchen is a Cupcake Decorating Station, and the basement is designated as the Use-All-The-Glitter-You-Want Area. Access to each of these zones requires a password. That password is only obtained if they eat their vegetables, which have been lightly steamed and arranged in a miniature replica of Disney World.

There is much glee and hooting. I try to wink at my parents conspiratorially, knowing that these noises are a harbinger to later meltdowns, that the kids don't yet realize they'll actually have to eat broccoli, but my parents don't wink back. They seem happy to have the chaos. I'm momentarily stunned, remembering the years they begged for quiet from my siblings and me, and then I remember we've only just arrived. Sometimes the noise takes a while to wear down one's resolve and/or sanity. They'll surely wink back tomorrow.

My husband, bolstered by the promise of twenty-four hours of uninterrupted thought, pulls me to the door.

"Come on, honey, let's let them have their time together."

"Do you need any last minute information? Routines? Favorite channels? Juice preferences?" I ask.

"If we need to know something, we'll ask the kids. Don't worry," my mother says while deftly braiding my daughter's usually uncooperative hair.

I look down at my daughter, who's enjoying having her hair played with. "Oh, you may notice that weird, crusty looking bruise thing over on the left side of her scalp . . . yeah, that's it," I say. "We're aware of it and probably heading to a doctor in a day or two if it doesn't improve. I don't like the look of it, so try not to touch it." My mother nods and keeps braiding, gently.

As my husband and I leave, the children run from room to room pulling out every toy and picking up every breakable, asking for snacks, hugs, TV, and if Grandpa will simultaneously play chess, checkers, poker, and soccer with them. It's the very definition of din. It's a level of noise that regularly causes me to raise my voice and insist on quiet tones and turn-taking, as was once requested of me.

Yet, now, here, my parents laugh and nod. "Yes!" they say. Yes to snacks, yes to TV, yes to everything.

Yes. The ultimate, decadent Grandparent Privilege.

The kids run in three directions, elated.

"Bye! I love you!" I call after them. No response.

My husband yells, "Kids! Say goodbye to your mother, or she won't leave."

They offer a joint "Bye" from the other room, too engrossed in something that has buzzers and buttons to inject much tone into their voices.

"Anything else?" my father asks, his hand already on the door ready to close it behind us.

Yes, I think. *They don't fall asleep easily, and we're still working on their table manners, and they fight a lot and, at some point, all that good behavior you've been able to bask in will melt off and, instead, there'll be a puddle of overtired children crying and screaming, and you can call me. Also, make sure they really have brushed their teeth when they say they have.*

"Just keep them alive," my husband says.

"Call me if you need to," I add.

"We've done this before," my dad says.

They'll be calling, I think as I hear my daughter insisting my mother watch her do the hula. My daughter, it should be noted, has never to my knowledge done the hula before.

***

I'm quiet as we get back in the car. My husband grabs my hand. "It's important they practice being away from us. And your folks can handle whatever our kids throw at them," he says.

I nod. As he turns the ignition, I double check my phone to make sure the ringer is switched on.

Moments after we get home, my husband flops on the couch and exhales. I sweep the floor, using the broom as a scraper in places where fruit snacks have been ground into the floor. When that's done, I start on the mound of laundry that has been doubling as an extra couch in the living room.

"You should stop and relax!" my husband says.

"Laundry doesn't stop." I don't know what to do with my time. I'd love to sit and knit or read, but I can't relax with a messy house, and that's what I have right now—a not so subtle reminder of three young lives being loudly lived to, if not their fullest, certainly their messiest.

He looks at me, wondering why I'm not enjoying the free time.

"I'm worried we overloaded my parents," I confess.

He's patient. "They've had the kids before," he reminds me.

"Not all three, not all at once, not overnight."

"What's the worst thing that could happen?" he asks.

"That they come back sugared up and with raised expectations about dietary laws and good parenting. And that my parents won't ever take them again," I say.

He shakes his head in surrender, closes his eyes, and falls asleep secure in the knowledge no child will come to opportunistically pounce on him for their own amusement. I stare at my phone. I know my parents and how easily frazzled they are—all I heard for eighteen years was how crazy I drove them, and I was a much better behaved small person than my children.

I decide to check in and, if need be, straighten out any behaviors. I can be the heavy, my parents can be the good guys, and the children can stay on the straight and narrow. Everyone wins. Everyone has a role to play.

My mother answers the call after one ring, just enough time for her to check the Caller ID. Her happy and high-pitched "Hello Mommy!" lets me know the kids are right there with her.

"Hi Mommy!" the kids echo in the background.

"Just checking in to make sure they're not in need of some course correction," I say.

"Oh, we're all doing so well," she's speaking for their benefit as much as mine. "The kids are helping make lunch and picking up their toys so they can go to the park."

I look over at the living room, which looks like Toys R Us came and threw a giant tantrum. I ask to speak to one of them. My mother puts my daughter on the phone.

"Grandma makes the best mac and cheese ever! And I'm eating broccoli! It's deeeelicious!" She sounds a lot happier than last night when she countered my presentation of broccoli with threats to call the police on me. I ask her to put Grandma back on the phone.

My mother gets back on the line. "Oh, I wanted to tell you—that scar on her head? It was just an old raisin that got stuck there and crusty, probably because you were afraid to wash it. It's gone now. Gotta go! Have fun! Enjoy the quiet!"

She hangs up, leaving me to accept the fact that I'll never need to craft a Parent of the Year Award acceptance speech.

The quiet affords me plenty of opportunity to worry. The calories from a big meal tend to launch my kids into hyperspace, so I'm sure my parents will need my intervention sooner rather than later.

I call an hour later, and, after four rings, my father answers.

"Yes?" *He* has obviously checked the Caller ID, too, and seems less than amused that I've called again. In the background, I hear the kids and my mom singing along to "Happy" by Pharrell Williams. Never in the four thousand times we've played that song, have they been okay with me singing along.

"Uh," I'm thrown by my father's impatience, as though he's willing to humor my intrusions for only so long.

"They're fine. Do you want to talk with them?" he asks, as though I thought they were in a hostage situation.

"Sure!" There's a click as he puts down the phone and calls my oldest and most chatty child to talk.

Without as much as a greeting, my first-born launches in. "Grandpa said when you were my age, you spilled a bottle of ink on his bed! Grandma makes the best chicken. We're going to the library and getting movies later! We get to watch them during dinner time. Grandma sweeps up the dog hair three times a day. Grandpa plays chess with us for hours!"

I look at my dog, who is asleep on my mop, and sigh. "Sounds like fun, honey. Please remember your manners and be helpful."

"Ok! Gotta go, they're starting the song over. Bye."

My jaw clenches. I clean some more, starting by chiseling giant blobs of toothpaste off the sinks, then by playing "What is making that smell" in my daughter's room. After addressing the fifteenth thank-you note from the boys' birthday party last week, I slam down the pen, exhausted from my day off from parenting.

My husband wakes up and suggests we start to think about dinner and a movie.

"Let me just check on my parents. It's witching hour. You know how hard it is right before dinner time." I pick up my phone and call. No answer. I try again. And again. I assume by now, my children have duct taped my parents to the kitchen table and are forcing them to listen to all the finer points of Minecraft. I tell my husband I need to go on a rescue mission.

***

I drive up to my parents' house, knowing I'll see the storm that has obviously been brewing in my children for weeks. They've been too excited for too long, the payoff today too great for them to hold it together. I know I'm needed.

Mere yards from my parents' house, I see a blur in the sky that I assume is a large bird. Then I see another. And another. I slow down. Those are no birds. My children are flying kites. Outside. They're all rosy cheeked and willingly wearing coats.

My parents look like I remember them looking thirty-five years ago. Engaged and energized. My mother spots me trying to drive off and waves—whether she's waving me off or waving me over, I can't tell. I wave back and keep driving, knowing the kids don't see me. Knowing they're fine. Knowing I'm ridiculous. Knowing that in some ways, I don't know my children or my parents very well.

I take out my phone and switch the ringer to vibrate, slipping it into my pocket where it stays for the rest of the evening, which I spend with my husband, talking about things other than our children and remembering that we have first names other than "Mom" and "Dad."

***

The next morning, I call one last time.

"Hi," my mother's voice is hoarse.

"Hi! Do you want me to come get them or do you want to keep them there a little longer? I promise . . . no more calls!"

There's a pause. "I think they miss you," she says. I hear someone crying in the background.

We head back to my folks' place, wondering exactly what we'll encounter, worried that it's exactly what we feared.

Again, my mother has sensed our arrival and opens the door before we get to the porch. "They didn't sleep well last night. It was hard for them to get to sleep after such an active day, but they were so excited to be here and to help me make breakfast that they bounced out of bed at five this morning!" Her triumphant smile is balanced by the shadows under her eyes.

She winks at me.

I wink back.

We call for the kids, who move much more slowly this morning. I don't immediately recognize them; they've been bathed so well. Even their cowlicks were happy to do as asked.

Goodbyes are sorrowful, filled with requests for more time, another sleepover, and one last treat. The hugs are sweet and real. Neither grandparent nor child wants to let go first.

We herd the children out the door.

I'm sure the click I heard wasn't the deadbolt. I'm also sure that what looked like my parents collapsing on the couch in a heap was just a figment of my imagination. I make a note to call them later—much later—to see if they'd like me to drop off dinner and a bottle of wine.

By the time I buckle my seatbelt, the children have started fighting, complaining, and seemed to have caught a cold. They are snapping at each other about windows and seat belts, asking if they can have screens, and why I don't do anything like Grandma.

Yet there's hope. I pop in a CD and the opening chords of "Happy" reverberate in the car. I begin to sing along, prompting groans. "Mom. Stop. Just stop." I do. They bicker, yawning, until they're too exhausted to determine who has trespassed into whose space in the cramped backseat. When my husband hits the brakes hard to avoid hitting an indecisive road squirrel, the children's suitcases again bonk them in the head. They all wail. But soon, they're all asleep, their beloved, innocent, clean faces are like cherubs.

And soon, too soon, I know, the Grandparent Privilege will be all mine.

Jackie Pick is a former teacher who is now writing her way through what she nervously identifies as her "second adolescence." Her writing has been featured on various parenting sites including Mamalode, The HerStories Project, and Scary Mommy, as well as the literary art magazine Selfish. *She is a contributing writer to* Multiples Illuminated *and to the HerStories Anthology,* So Glad They Told Me. *Jackie is the co-creator and co-writer of the upcoming short film* Bacon Wrapped Dates *and occasionally performs sketch and musical comedy in Chicago. When she's not in one of her three children's school pick-up lanes, she can be found on Twitter (@ jackiepick) apologizing for not updating her blog (jackiepickauthor.com).*

PEDICURE WITH DAD
By Ashley Collins

The slender, young Vietnamese woman tugged my hand forward and forced my gaze back to her fingers, where she was in the process of cutting my cuticles.

I'd been staring at my dad, who was getting his feet massaged in a pedicure chair to my left. His blue eyes were closed and the expression on his face was one of utter bliss, like that of my dog when I scratch her belly. I was grateful he could enjoy this moment in the shitstorm his life had become since being diagnosed with acute myeloid leukemia three months ago. He was still active and fit at 78, playing his regular games of golf and tennis. There were no signs yet of the cancer weakening him. It was hard to believe those sinister cells were now flowing through his blood, a promise of death coming too early. I wasn't ready.

I turned back around to look at my dad and tried to will love into the hands of the pedicurist working on his feet. Ton, the nail technician (my dad had asked his name earlier), was deftly cutting and filing my dad's thick, horny toenails. Even when I was a child, his toenails were yellowed and curving, in ugly prehistoric contrast to his dark handsomeness. Now, Ton held what looked like a cheese grater in his gloved hands, and to my horror, he began to swipe it across the callouses on my dad's feet. Chemotherapy had made his blood thin, and I worried the sharpness of the utensil might start him bleeding.

When Ton put down the grater and picked up a pumice stone, I exhaled in relief and then turned around to inspect my own short and peeling nails. I'd picked off most of the gel polish a few days before in a moment of nervous agitation, but putty-colored stains still stubbornly clung to the outer edges. The manicurist was trying to buff them smooth, but the damage was done. I hoped my dad's blood was stronger than my nails.

My 17-year-old daughter sat at a manicure station in front of me. I took in her slumped shoulders, the long, blond hair hanging halfway down her back in a tangled wave, and felt a rush of fierce love for her. It was fitting she was with us, because although my dad adored all of his grandchildren, he shared a special bond with this child of mine.

She loved him completely and steadfastly, as only the young can the old, without reservation or baggage. The generation between them seemed to have eliminated all judgment and expectation. They could tease each other unmercifully, sharing the same prank-like sense of humor. In the long months between visits, they argued by text over who was ahead by more games in backgammon.

But I think my dad was drawn to my daughter because he recognized that her steady nature was an antidote to the fear and worry that plagued him. Not fear for himself, not even about dying, but fear for those he loved. I could see that my daughter's old soul somehow soothed him. She had that effect on me, too, as she balanced gracefully in the eye of the storm our family created, unafraid of strong emotions. I allowed myself to be comforted by her presence.

The sound of my dad's giggle pulled my attention back to his chair, where his foot involuntarily jerked away from Ton's hand holding the pumice stone. My dad had always been ticklish. "Sorry, sorry," he apologized sheepishly to Ton, catching my eye and grinning. "Ton owns this place with his wife and sister!" he said to me loudly, and almost proudly, from across the salon. "They're from Danang!" I smiled back at him, nodding. My daughter turned around in her chair at the sound of his raised voice, her mouth curving up slightly in comedic indulgence. Her rules forbidding embarrassing behavior clearly did not apply to him. She caught my eye, and the look she gave me seemed to melt away the years and roles between us.

Dad was asking Ton all sorts of questions about his life, in a voice loud enough for the whole salon to hear. I heard him tell Ton about the trip he and my mother had taken to Vietnam several years before, as if that were connection enough to get personal. My dad had never been inside a nail salon, and I could tell he was fascinated. He'd always been curious about people's stories and adept at ferreting them out. It was a quality I admired now, although when I was my daughter's age, it had embarrassed me greatly.

Dad could start up a conversation with anyone, in any circumstance. He'd learn about their hopes and dreams and then feel compelled to help them. The busboy at the Mexican restaurant, where we ate once a week for years, ended up going to community college at my dad's urging and having a career in restaurant management. A woman who worked at my dad's office couldn't get a mortgage, so he introduced her to his private banker. There were countless times he left me picking up tennis balls with the heavy metal basket to help the person on the tennis court next to us, because he believed he could improve their stroke with a few simple changes.

I felt a range of emotions between complete mortification and jealous pique in those moments his attention was diverted, but when I grew up, I realized he just couldn't resist helping people.

And he helped me plenty. He taught me how to play tennis, to ski, to ride a bike. When I tried out for softball in middle school, he spent many evenings before dinner playing catch with me in the dusky twilight. The thwack of the ball hitting my mitt punctuated his instructions on my throwing motion, how to position my glove to catch. His praise when I did it correctly was enthusiastic. "Thaaaat's it!" he'd call across the gloaming.

He played horse with me at the basketball hoop behind our garage, taught me how to shoot a free throw, dribble with my left hand so I could do a layup from both sides. He taught me how to play ping-pong and to water ski. He taught me how to train a hunting dog and how to walk carrying a shotgun. When I was 11, he taught me how to load and fire that gun. "Widen your stance. Now bend your knees slightly, cheek firm against the barrel, and hold the butt tight into your shoulder," he'd advise, so I wouldn't get bruised. "Now say 'pull,'" he instructed me.

"Pull!" I called, and he swung his arm in a wide arc, releasing the clay pigeon into the air in front of me from the spring-loaded launcher.

He taught me how to cast a fly rod on the lawn before taking me to the river, where we sat for hours waiting for the fish to rise. I didn't really care if I caught anything, but I loved being near him and hearing the sound of the water gurgling, while ducks floated and flapped and squawked on the surface. Canadian geese flew over our heads in big V-formations, their calls adding to the natural symphony of that corner of the Pacific Northwest.

But my dad didn't just teach me about the outdoors and sports. He also taught me how to play poker and gin rummy, backgammon, and chess, to think logically and to strategize, to be bold. Many nights he had me read out loud to him, so that I'd learn to enunciate properly and be comfortable with public speaking. He pushed me hard academically, encouraged me to excel in whatever I tried. Competition was valued highly by my dad, as a method to improve. Sometimes it broke us apart, my brothers and me, but it also gave us grit. I learned early that I couldn't always win, and that I'd better be a good sport when I lost, or I wouldn't get to play again. Out of all the skills and values he taught me, though, my favorite was the art of storytelling.

As the manicurist firmly massaged my hands, my eyes started to fill with tears like water rising in a tank. Her therapeutic touch was melting the thin sheet of ice I had frozen around my heart to protect it. I blinked carefully so the tears wouldn't spill, wishing I could apply nail polish to harden my heart as easily as the young Vietnamese woman did to my nails. I wasn't ready to lose my dad.

Ashley Collins is mother to three grown children and currently lives in Connecticut with the pets they left behind. She graduated from Stanford University in 1987 with a B.A. in Anthropology. She has traveled extensively, living in New York City, London, and Seattle prior to moving to Connecticut. Her work has appeared online at Grown and Flown, Horse Network, the Roar Sessions and in the Band of Women anthology Nothing But The Truth So Help Me God: 73 Women on Life's Transitions. *She currently writes a blog about her family and animals, and is working on a memoir about mothers and daughters and horses. She also competes as an equestrian show jumper. You can read more about her at ashleycollinswriter.com and on social media at facebook.com/ashleycollinswriter and instagram.com/ashleygriffincollins.*

I CAN'T GO BACK, BUT I CAN ALWAYS REMEMBER
By Rudri Bhatt Patel

For twenty-seven years, I spent my days and nights in one place. My mother, father, sister, and I called it home. Most evenings we gathered at our brown dining table to eat buttery *roti,* spice-infused *dal,* and curried veggies. A mixture of coconut and saffron percolated through the house while the TV played the latest episode of *Wheel of Fortune.* The melding of our Indian heritage and American life created the arc of our personal landscape in a small Texan town. The table and our home became a metaphorical bridge to negotiate the differences.

On this chipped mahogany table, I spent many nights deciphering statistics or writing my senior paper on Jane Austen's *Pride and Prejudice.* My father stayed up with me and made his famous cinnamon-infused coffee. After brewing it the old fashioned way, he poured it from one container to another, creating a creamy froth and said, "Who needs Starbucks?" On Sundays, we gathered in our living room and prepared for our weekly Dallas Cowboys game by eating subs and chips and drinking our favorite soda.

Our house witnessed milestones too numerous to count.

I learned, with my father's help, to ride my bike and car down our street. One night my teenage hormones called all the shots and propelled me to run away from home. As I sprinted down our street, my father's car followed my every step. After I dawdled for forty minutes, it made sense to just get back into the car and return home. I boomeranged there for most of my life—I found my safe place, even if I didn't readily acknowledge it at the time.

Those crème-black bricks held so many of my stories. If the bricks could have a conversation, they'd tell you about my nervous anxiety when my then-boyfriend-now-husband picked me up on the front porch for our date. My husband met my parents for the first time in my childhood living room. I still recall my mom's colorful *sari*, my father's cream dress shirt, and my blue and black cinched dress and how we exchanged a flurry of words, a potpourri of English and *Gujarati* filling the air. After we married and had our daughter, there were numerous visits to her grandparents' home, my childhood home. It was the place where my daughter shared memories with her grandpa—he tickled her arm until she chuckled her raucous belly laugh, chased her around the living room, and helped her with her alphabet.

***

The house cried along with us when my father passed away in my childhood bedroom. The windows witnessed his body being placed inside the black hearse on a dark March night. We watched him leave forever from the front porch. We reluctantly embraced his return as a box, his ashes packed away like a gift.

Now, years later, I can't go back to that place to reminisce anymore.

My childhood home belongs to another family now. When I visit, I do so as an outsider. The table still inhabits the space but with a new set of names. As much as I hope the space will offer great memories for this family, I still feel my father and my childhood as part of the ether in the room. The place that served as a meeting ground for so many connections and memories will no longer serve as my safe harbor. For so many years, the house and the table inside weren't objects, but real people in all our lives, witnessing joys, sadness, and every other emotion, big or small.

What reconciles the space between mourning and living?

***

The mountains dot the horizon; the light and shadow create its own landscape as the sun splatters golden coins on the grey pavement. I reach down, tie my shoelaces, and adjust my headphones to my favorite running music station. One foot in front of the other, I move through my run, alternating between sprints and a leisurely walk.

In my path, I notice an elderly Indian man with a long-sleeve checkered shirt, black pants, and a brown beanie that covers his forehead. His pace is slow, but methodical. We exchange a cursory glance, I smile, and he nods his head. A few seconds later, a single tear rolls down my cheek.

To no one in particular, I mouth the words, "Oh goodness, he looks so much like Dad." My father loved his walks, his preferred way to meditate. Intersecting with this stranger, the familiar brimmed to the surface.

"I miss him so much." This time I pause in the middle of my run to let this statement percolate in a way I sometimes suppress. Why does this still happen? It has been seven years since Dad's passing. Why do the torrent of tears spill out like I'm acknowledging this loss for the first time?

I've questioned my grief—cross-examining it like a hostile witness on the stand. Why can't I get it together? Why does the grief come unexpectedly like an errant meteor in the sky? Shouldn't it be over by now?

With the questions, sometimes epiphanies arrive. I've given myself permission to cry in the middle of the grocery store when I see butterscotch ice cream (my father's favorite), when I run across a quote by John F. Kennedy (a president my father adored), and even when there isn't a triggering memory but the grief surfaces nonetheless.

Grief is one's own. And it isn't meant to be judged.

The embers of grief do not have a timeline. The pathway is one that cannot be managed, much like my morning runs. When dawn breaks, I slide into my shoes and run as if I know what I will encounter. The truth—my jog follows the same route with the familiar street signs, but each run is different because of what I witness in the periphery. Sometimes a rabbit serves as my companion; other times I side-step a lady walking her brown Labrador, or I might make room for serious bicyclists racing down the road.

It's an apt metaphor for grief—the unpredictable way of learning to live without someone who anchored my life for so many decades. I've stopped analyzing the why's of my tears and I accept the unexpected sadness, claiming it without the expectation that when I wipe the last tear from my face, I won't feel melancholy anymore.

The sorrow and the reminders twist sometimes toward the goodness of the memories I shared with my father— the afternoons at the local ice-cream store, the evenings debating the latest political candidates at our kitchen table, and the friendship I shared with him.

I'm so grateful I rejected adhering to some arbitrary timeline on my grief.

With a deep breath, finishing my jog, I turn the corner, thinking of the elderly man, and one thought crosses my mind—maybe, it's my father's way of saying *hello*.

I can't go back, but I can always remember.

Rudri Bhatt Patel is an attorney turned writer and editor. Prior to attending law school, she graduated with an M.A. in English with an emphasis in creative writing. Her work has appeared in the Washington Post; *Brain, Child Magazine; Role Reboot; The Review Review; Huffington Post; Literary Mama; Mamalode and elsewhere. She writes her personal musings on her site, www.beingrudri. com, and is currently working on a memoir that explores Hindu culture, grief and appreciating life's ordinary graces.*

TO CALL YOU MAMA
By Chelsea Schott

I met you on a Saturday, a day Mama had taken off work. You were late, which was something I was to learn about you—time revolved around you. You set it so. I'd waited for hours to take your hand in my own, my eyes to meet yours, to study your face for recognizable family details. Would I see some of my own face in yours? I was 8 years old when you entered the room. I could smell your perfume and feel my own heartbeat in the back of my throat. I'd been carefully prepped to call you only by your first name. It was one of your rules, and there were many. I didn't mind.

My grandmother: thick German accent, black hair, and no concept of time.

Rita.

Two weeks later, I heard your name again on the lips of Mama. It'd be the last time she'd say your name for years. You had a way with time, and most of it was spent apart from us.

On a Friday in January, when I was no longer a child, you sat at your husband's funeral. Even though he was my grandfather, I called him "Daddy" like everyone did, and I loved him more than I loved you. You arrived that day in a car by yourself, and as I passed through family members speaking in low tones and hushed sentences over the open casket of my grandfather, my fingers trembled inside my coat pockets when I saw you. I watched you cry into a handkerchief and tuck his military flag close to your chest, as if you could hold his full military career in your hands.

I knew you lived in another town, in another life, and wanted more. I wanted more too: to know more about who you were. I wanted to know your secrets, all of them. Mama shushed me, ended my questioning between cigarette smoke-filled sighs in the car. "Rita was my mother," she said. "She left when I was 13 years old. Here one day, gone the next."

Three days after my fifteenth birthday, you sent me a card with one hundred dollars in it. It was more money than I'd ever seen, more money than Mama had. I locked my bedroom door, lay on my bed and studied your penmanship, the funny way you crossed your sevens, and I stared into the stern face of Franklin on the bill. What did his eyes see before you tucked him into that pale pink envelope? Your address read, "Wichita Falls, Texas." I hid the card under my mattress.

In my seventeenth birthday card, dated September 2nd, your note said, "Jean says that giving you one hundred dollars is spoiling you and that is too much money for any child to have—have a Happy Birthday, Love your grandmother, Rita." I had no idea who Jean was, and that year I didn't buy new clothes for school.

When I was a freshman in college, I picked up the phone, dialed the operator, and got your home number. Saturdays became our calling days. I sat silent as you unraveled your life's stories to me: who you were, where you came from, why you left, and why you stayed. Your history is my history, too. I loved your advice on men and money—which to keep and which to cultivate. When it came to both, you told me, "It helps if you're pretty."

You were more correct than I could've ever known. But I was poor and single and could do the math. You were the pretty one, you always had been. I sent you photos, cards, mementoes, and forgave any wrong, because you were my grandmother. You were a piece of me. It was the first time I loved you.

On a Friday night, walking home to the dorm, I found a box marked, "Free Shit." Inside were two sweaters (one purple, one blue), some textbooks, an overnight bag, and a new leather satchel. Obviously, the remnants of an ex-girlfriend's belongings tossed out by an angry lover—*such are the ways of college romances*—at least, I imagined them so. This ex-girlfriend was my size, at least in sweaters, so I took the box home.

The satchel was brand new with gold hardware still wrapped in tissue paper. I ran my fingers over the leather-bound Dooney & Bourke. It was nicer than anything I owned. I could return it or, perhaps, sell it and buy groceries. My eyes hovered over the carefully manicured stitching; the new, stiff leather; the earthy, rawhide smell.

I carefully wrapped the tissue paper back over the bag and boxed it up. The next day, I rushed to the university post office. I mailed it to you fully aware that I did so with the impulse of a child.

The kind of child who plucks flowers in handfuls for Mama.

***

On a Sunday, when I was a senior in college in the depths of a wintry February, Mama's voice erupted through my answering machine, its tones conveyed concern and panic. We drove to your farm house and found you living alone. No heat, no food. Your mind was confused. You couldn't remember to pay the gas bill, but you could remember to buy more cat food. You couldn't recall where you left your paperwork but carefully cataloged years of junk mail. We moved you and all of your things—bags of papers, years of mail, boxes of trash—to another home. Mama's eyes moved to mine; we said things no one else could hear—*Rita needs help.*

In the garage, I found Daddy's lunch box and winter hat. I pressed the hat to my face, inhaling deeply, desperately, trying to pick up his scent; although I knew

I'd long forgotten his scent. I thought enough time had passed, but it hadn't. I cried. Hard.

And when I packed your things that were mostly trash, I found a box still wrapped in shiny, but faded, pink paper. The label read, "To: Rita, Happy Valentines, Love, Daddy." I ripped it open anyway to find an unopened Chanel No. 5 bottle still wrapped, still intact. You never even cared to open the gift, and the perfume completely evaporated. In this moment, I hated you as my eyes welled over.

I hated you on this Sunday because of all the Sundays you threw away with my grandfather, with my mother, with me. I hated you for all the gifts you ignored, all the birthdays you missed, all the Christmas mornings you spent with God-knows-who instead of us. I hated you for all the anniversaries and celebrations you forgot, the ones you got wrong, and the ones you didn't give a damn about anyway. I hated you for all the gifts of love you tossed aside that collected with the trash.

I hated you for all the evaporated bottles.

In the same room as the Chanel, I found a bag of department store makeup. The kind in little, mint-green boxes with gold lettering and tissue paper. The kind scented with heavy perfume I could smell through the box. I knew you bought these for yourself. You walked across the shiny tiled floor in the pretty downtown department store, your heels clicking through the wide aisles, and you leaned on the glass counter trying on a new shade of lipstick, staring into your own mouth in the close-up mirror. You pressed your lips together and blotted them on the tissue the saleslady offered. You paid with cash, check, or a hundred credit cards from money that came from God-knows-where. And you tossed this new purchase on your vanity with your dozens of colognes and creams and jewelry boxes and tiny jeweled-framed photos of yourself. I knew you did that.

And while I should've been joining Mama in pity and planning your new home, I didn't. I stepped into the hallway and made sure I was alone. You stood in the dining room talking with the movers, and I unzipped my backpack and stuffed all your pretty makeup inside. Bag, tissue paper and all.

***

Around Christmas that same year, the calls started. You called Mama. You called me. In the middle of the night, you accused us of stealing your money and taking your cars. We worried more. I stopped calling on Saturdays and weeknights. We couldn't stop you from calling us. Whether you wanted us or not, we're yours.

I sent a card in March, and when my son was born, I sent a picture. You didn't respond. In late September, three years later, when I finally found myself on your doorstep, you didn't know who I was anymore.

And I may not have ever known you.

That same month, Mama moved you into her home. And for the first time, I heard her call you "Mama," and my skin tensed knowing you weren't anyone's Mama and didn't deserve the title. Your paperwork piled on Mama's kitchen table and littered the countertop: years of bank accounts, insurance, deeds, property titles and claims, passports and photos of you—the most gorgeous thing I'd ever seen, black, beautiful eyes staring through a 1953 passport.

"Mama."

She said it again and again. She loved you despite all your faults and failures. Loved you when I couldn't, when I wouldn't. Cared for you like she would a child. Cared for you the way you should've cared for her.

I looked at your face, now wrinkled and withered, your once-black curls streaked with white, your shoulders hunched, delicate, your arthritic hands weaved together with veins as thick as yarn crocheted over bony fingers. Your thin frame underneath a sweater with ridiculously overdressed jewels sewn on the front; surely something Mama bought for you. Something she'd seen in a store, picked off the rack, held up for a better view, decided she liked it, decided it reminded her of you. I stared too long, and you cast one of those sideways glances toward me—*the kind of glance that reads thoughts*—and I felt ashamed.

I felt embarrassed by my own face. Shamed and humiliated. What did I know of love?

In the summertime, Mama called me. She was exhausted by you. You were demanding, angry, and haughty. You demanded to go home, you insisted on driving, you refused to tip the waitress, the hairdresser, the grocery boy. You slapped the sitter—the third one in a week. Mama didn't ask me for help, she never would. Guilt doesn't allow us that privilege of thinking we deserve a moment to ourselves, to watch a movie with friends, or have a glass of wine on a Saturday afternoon. Guilt, instead, taunts us from within, *"Didn't she change your diapers, too?"*

I picked you up for a weekend stay. You wore your oversized sunglasses and navy cardigan, even though it was ninety-five degrees outside. You also insisted on bringing your five checkbooks. We listened to Handel's "Messiah" for the entire forty-minute drive, because it made you smile and that made me smile, too. Your hands conducting, you leaned out the window to conduct to the highway traffic, and we all laughed.

When you saw my three-bedroom, two-bath, two-car garage brick home, you called it a "dump" and asked, "Who lives here?" I laughed it off and let you into the guest room—my stepdaughter's princess-themed bedroom with bunk beds. After dinner, I helped you into your nightgown and you started to cry. You missed home, you hated it here, you hated it there at Mom's. I feared I let you drink too much wine, and I had. You soon slept it off, and I felt the great release of weight from tired relief, like a worn-out new mother when her infant finally rests.

At four o'clock in the morning, my husband found you in the dew-soaked grass of our backyard, under a warm, July night buzzing with mosquitoes and junebugs. You were wearing only your panties and seemed to be talking to the trees. We brought you in, dressed you, and put you back to bed.

You asked me who I was. I answered, "Mama."

***

In May, Mama went to your house in Wichita Falls, the house on Call Field Road, and split the remainder of your earthly possessions between my sister and me. A week later, a truck arrived at my house loaded with box after box of European artifacts: a lifetime of possessions, of memories not my own. My house filled with crystal, Bavarian gold-lined dishes, Tiffany glass, Romanian silver, tea cups and saucers, military awards, silver chalices engraved with my grandfather's name, shelves of German Hummel figurines, half a dozen cuckoo clocks and walls of oil paintings from France, Austria, and Italy.

In one of the boxes, I found a vaguely familiar parcel, addressed in my own handwriting. Inside, the Dooney & Bourke green leather bag I'd given you, tissue still on the hardware. Untouched.

My own evaporated bottle.

I was exhausted by the dust, the history. My rooms filled with the belongings of a woman I didn't know, I could never know, a woman whose secrets would become my own.

A week later, Mama showed me the photos she found. Your life before her. Your first husband—a family we never knew. And a photo that arrests us all: your arms wrapped lovingly around a young boy. Your cheek against his, smiling into the camera—his unmistakable eyes—a mirror image reflection of your own unmistakable eyes.

How many of us did you walk away from?

You have more secrets than I ever wanted to know. More than I could ever forget.

I don't know whether to love you or not.

Most Sundays, we visited you in the nursing home. Sometimes you smiled, sometimes you didn't. Some weeks I visited, some weeks I didn't. You didn't dance with the other old folks when they played forties music, you didn't exercise when the nurse gave you hand weights, and you damn sure didn't let them feed you with a spoon or give you a bath. You couldn't remember my name or your own, but you knew who you *were* and who you *weren't.*

When you'd see us come in the door, you'd turn away and frown. You didn't speak anymore, but you didn't have to either. I had to push, nudge, and threaten my older children to hug you, to kiss your cheek. I'd whisper to them between clenched teeth, "Get over there *now* and hug Grandma!" They had no understanding of age or death, no realization that bodies breakdown, joints swell, skin wrinkles, hands shake. On the brink of adolescence, anticipating adulthood, unaware of life's progression and end, my children could neither imagine their own decay nor accept it: the smells of the aged, the sight of grown men in diapers, women curled up like fetuses in wheelchairs, all sleeping under a blasting TV.

I was ashamed of them in those moments, embarrassed of their refusal to embrace you—maybe it's something I taught them. For every time we drove past the nursing home and didn't stop, for all the years when I was two weeks late in remembering your birthday, when I cut short our visit because I had pressing matters at home, when I considered our visits with you as an entry on a to-do list of petty tasks during my busy day, maybe somehow I taught them to diminish their respect for you.

Maybe I was ashamed of myself in your presence.

My kids' whining questions rang out as if you were deaf: "When are we leaving?" "Can we go out to eat?"

"Could you drop us off at the mall?"

My baby girl mounted your wheelchair, grabbed fistfuls of your sweater, and crawled up in your lap. You swatted her away like a fly, and I had to laugh, because sometimes I wanted to do that, too.

At nine o'clock on a Tuesday, you had another seizure. *Or was it a stroke? Who the hell knows?* You didn't wake up this time. Mama tried to give you crushed ice, only because she wanted so badly for you to do something normal like sit up and swallow and say, "Good morning." Something more than what you were doing. What we all knew you were doing—dying.

So, I picked up two misting spray bottles from the corner drugstore to wet your dry mouth. To give you moisture, water, a drink, a kiss. So you could swallow again. One pink, one green, for no particular reason at all. And when I checked out, the girl behind the register said, "Merry Christmas."

I'd forgotten what day it was. And I knew the world was moving on past you already, past me, too.

The nurse hated my idea about the mist, shook her head from side to side, and gave me a bowl of cool water with tiny pink sponges. The kind with little sticks, the kind used to comfort the dying. The back of the sponge package read: "To assist those in various states of compromised consciousness."

I dipped the little pink sponge in the bowl, letting it swell with cool water to wet your lips, like vinegar given to Jesus on the cross. I slid the bloated sponge from side to side, caressing the enamel of your teeth, setting it so gently on your tongue, and you bit down and swallowed. I did this for hours.

Because I had to do *something.*

When Mama went home for dinner, I stayed. I prayed for you to live, I prayed for you to die easily; I didn't believe God was listening anyway. And I hoped you would speak, sit up, clear that rattle from your chest.

Swat me away like a fly.

I tipped the priest after he read your last rites and gave him all the money I had: crumpled up bills from my wallet, from my coat pocket, and from the tiny pocket in my purse. Tens, ones, twenties. I don't know why, I just did it, even when he tried to refuse. Even when I couldn't see through my own tears.

When the sun set, and your bowl of water was nearly empty, I stayed by your bed. Combing your hair, because I knew you'd want that. I picked out another nightgown for you, the baby blue one with lace at the wrists. I stroked your forehead—the skin was so smooth there—and held your hand. And when you quieted your breathing and relaxed, I pressed my mouth to your ear, inhaling the scent of your hair through my weeping, and kissed you one last time.

On New Year's Day, we buried you next to Daddy. At your funeral, we all commented on your beauty. Even years later, as we look at photographs, we are stunned by your full lips, black ringlets of hair, and eyes that stare us down, daring us to look elsewhere, knowing damn well we can't. You chose for yourself the flashiest coffin I'd ever seen. The same kind I'd surely choose for myself.

***

Days, weeks later, as the March snow begins to melt in wide patches across the red, muddy earth, you still reside in my brain, permeating the grey matter of thought, extracting things I can't even mention out loud or to myself. I think I see you everywhere. Passing strangers, crowds of people; every face looks like yours.

Maybe I'm afraid at how similar we really are. How our lives have traced the same steps, the same paths, the same missteps. I see Mama in myself, too, and am ashamed, guilt-ridden for reasons I cannot fathom.

***

On a Saturday, deep in June when it's too hot, too early, I'm alone. Distracted in a mundane task, I stumble across your photo. My mind finds you at rest in the ground again; the nagging alarm of loss interred deep into the earth of my brain reminds me of the grief and separation. Yet, I sense your voice saying that little phrase you used to say, dragging out each word: "You really have no idea, darling," always exaggerating your losses. And, I whisper in reply, "Yes, Mama. I really didn't have any idea, did I?"

It is in this moment, the moment I "hear" your voice, that I release all the doubt, all the accusations for no reason at all.

My lips part and whisper the name again and again: "Mama."

Its release so easy, so simple. My pardon not for you, but for myself. I feel something break wide open, something pass over—that hot June day. As my eyes well at the sight of your picture, I must admit, I really have no idea about anything. My fingers tremble to hold your picture, to meet your eyes. I swallow back the pain in my throat, the longing to say to you with shaking voice:

"Yes, Mama, yes."

Chelsea Schott is a writer living in Houston, Texas. A recent graduate of Rice University and a regular contributor to the Houston Press, she divides her time between teaching writing craft and writing on contemporary music culture. You can find her work in such publications as Under the Gum Tree, Winter Tangerine Review, Texas Music Magazine, Germ Magazine, *and the anthology,* My Other Ex *by the Her Stories Publishers.*

THE BLUE ROOM
By Jill Wilbur Smith

I had wanted to paint the room, but there wasn't time. My mother-in-law's decline happened quickly. One day my husband, Gary, was taking her to Target to get her own groceries—a week later, the phone call came in the middle of the night that she'd fallen out of bed and couldn't get up.

So we moved her into our youngest daughter's old bedroom. The blue wall, chosen by Sarah when she was 14, stayed as it was. I wonder what my 91-year-old mother-in-law, Doris, thought as she lay on her deathbed, watching the blue wall change as the November sun slanted through the window.

I could've painted the wall two years earlier when Sarah moved away, but I wasn't ready then. I wanted the reminder of my creative child, the girl who'd selected the bright blue paint and had chosen to only paint one wall with the trendy hue. I wanted to remember the independent young woman who'd packed everything from her room into her car and moved to another state less than a week after her high school graduation, leaving my husband and me with an empty nest.

Now there wasn't time to paint the wall, because

there were too many other things to do. Gary arranged for hospice to deliver a hospital bed and a wheelchair to our home. He interviewed nursing agencies to provide supplemental care and to give him a break from being the primary caregiver.

I went to work, escaping the house for nine hours a day and thinking about things other than the woman trying to die in my spare bedroom. Gary stayed at home with her because he could, because this was the time we'd prepared for when we agreed he'd leave the workforce to pursue his writing career.

After work, I took over. Bringing her dinner. Helping her change her pajamas. Standing outside the bathroom door as she struggled to wash her face and brush her teeth, determined to maintain these small daily habits when everything else in her life was no longer in her control.

In my limited spare time, I started the process of moving her things out of her apartment. She insisted on going through her clothes and choosing what she wanted to keep. I brought her clothes to our house, filling two closets and four large suitcases with the designer blouses and slacks I knew she'd never wear again.

All the while, she lay helpless in my second-floor bedroom, fearful I'd give something away without her knowledge. I got her approval on every piece of furniture and sat by her bedside at night holding her hand, assuring her I hadn't left anything in the dresser drawers. Finally, I took pictures of every empty drawer and cabinet, showing them to her to calm her fears.

I hired movers to move her personal belongings and a few pieces of furniture to our house. I brought her favorite chair and ottoman into the blue room along with her desk and a nightstand. I tried to make the room familiar and comfortable for her. Still, the blue glared behind the TV, a constant reminder that once again she'd been displaced from all that was familiar to her.

***

We'd never planned to be my mother-in-law's caregivers. In fact, we'd moved twelve hundred miles away from her and my father-in-law more than two decades earlier. We'd always assumed they'd live out their years in their New Orleans home until they were too old to care for themselves. Then they'd live with my husband's sister, Lesley. But Hurricane Katrina forced them from New Orleans. My father-in-law passed away and then, unexpectedly, so did Lesley. So Doris came to live near us.

I always had a good relationship with my mother-in-law, but I never let myself get too close. I wasn't her daughter and didn't have the same type of relationship with her that she had with her three children. She once told me, "Anyone who hurts my children is nothing to

me. You hurt my children, you're out of my life forever."
I don't think she meant to direct the comment at me, but I
took it to heart. I had no thoughts of ever hurting her son,
but she made it very clear where I'd stand if I did.

From that day, I put up a protective barrier. I only let
myself get so close, never seeking her approval so she
couldn't hurt me if she criticized my choices. I wasn't her
child and thought, then, that I'd never be viewed as such
by her. This was never clearer to me than when my father-
in-law passed away, and my name was omitted from his
obituary. Only Gary and the girls were listed. Unlike my
children, who were related to the family by blood, my
only bond was a marriage certificate, a piece of paper
that Doris had learned through experience could easily be
dissolved. Perhaps she also put up a barrier, not wanting
to get too close to me in case I left her son, the way three
men had previously abandoned her two daughters.

But when she moved to live near us, things changed.
She'd lost her daughter, the most heartbreaking pain I
could imagine. Her other daughter was unable to care for
her at the time. My oldest daughter, Emily, had just left for
college, and I understood the pain of separation. So I tried
to fill the void.

For six years, I was the dutiful daughter-in-law. We
brought her to our house for Sunday dinner every week.
Gary drove her to the grocery store and to the doctor's

office. I took her to the shopping mall and visited with her in the senior living apartment complex where she lived four miles from our home. Friends told me I was a saint, questioned why I did so much for her. I couldn't understand their questions. It never felt like enough to me.

I didn't call Doris every day like her daughter did. But then that wasn't what I was used to. If I was lucky, I talked to my college-aged daughter a few times a month. I only called my own mother once a week. Perhaps it was the guilt I felt from being six hundred miles away from my mother, leaving the burden of her care to my sisters. I'd moved far away from my parents, leaving Michigan for New Orleans shortly after I graduated from college.

After Emily was born, we moved to Minnesota, closer, but still twelve hours away. Moving to Minnesota meant depriving both my parents *and* my in-laws of the close proximity to their children and grandchildren. When Doris moved to Minnesota, I felt I had the chance to make up for that decision. I tried to pack her final years with all of the daily experiences we both had missed during the nearly two decades we'd lived apart. I tried to be the type of daughter I knew my mother wanted me to be.

Six weeks after we moved Doris in to live with us, after all of her care had been planned, after the apartment had been packed up and moved out and cleaned, after we turned our house upside down to accommodate not only my mother-in-law but also the daily health care workers and constant visitors, her daughter, Karen, arrived from Louisiana.

In an instant, I felt like I was being replaced. It suddenly didn't seem to matter that I'd been the one at Doris' side during the multiple hospital stays and lengthy rehabilitation following her first surgery. It seemed insignificant that it'd been me who'd listened when the doctor said "cancer," who'd taken the call in the middle of the night when the pain from pancreatitis required paramedics to take Doris to the hospital.

Her "real" daughter was by her side now. I was grateful that Karen could be with her mother during her final days. But I couldn't help feeling like I'd just been marking time for the past six years, filling in for someone else. Karen insisted she be the one to sit vigil with her mother, relieving me of the burden. She thanked me for everything I'd done for "her family." I know she acted from a generous place, but it felt like I was being dismissed.

The U.S. government reinforced in me the feeling I was an outsider. I wanted to take time off work under the Family and Medical Leave Act (FMLA), but in-laws don't qualify for protection under the law. I'm fortunate my work gave me all of the flexibility I needed even without the federal mandate, but I was still hurt by the realization that even the government didn't think I was enough.

On the Sunday after she arrived, Karen made one of Doris' favorite meals—homemade jambalaya—from Doris' recipe. While Karen was cleaning the kitchen, I fed Doris the rice and sausage. I was afraid it would upset her stomach, but I wasn't willing to stop spooning the rice into her mouth every time she muttered, "more." I wished my blue room were a time machine that could take her back to her carefree days in New Orleans when she was a young bride gallivanting around town on my father-in-law's arm.

"Where do you want to pretend we are?" I asked.

"La Cuisine," she whispered. She closed her eyes, and I put another bite in her mouth.

"Remember the year we had Thanksgiving dinner there?" I asked.

She nodded. "More."

"Let's pretend this is that nice sauvignon blanc you and Dad used to like," I said as I held the ice water to her lips. She smiled as she sipped through the straw.

I closed my eyes, too, and tried to imagine we were back in one of our favorite New Orleans restaurants, the smell of shrimp and crawfish wafting through the air. Or maybe we could be transported to The Blue Room, the supper club at the Roosevelt Hotel. It was her favorite haunt in the early days of her marriage. She and my father-in-law would dress in their Sunday best to go eat decadent food and drink fine wine while listening to the smooth, rhythmic jazz sounds of Pete Fountain or Al Hirt. The Blue Room was where she first ate lobster. It embodied everything she loved about New Orleans.

I wish I could've done more to make her feel at home, although I don't know that it was even possible. No amount of paint or food or photographs could transform a suburban Minnesota house into New Orleans of the sixties. All I could do was make her comfortable so that her memories could transport her home.

As the sun began to set, Doris finally turned her head away as I lifted the spoon to her mouth. I'd given her enough. She didn't want any more. It'd be the last time she ate anything. It'd be the last real conversation we'd have.

I wasn't alone with Doris again until the moments right after she died a week later. Gary had left the house for the first time in days. Karen had taken a break and was crocheting in the family room. I was working from home, because we knew the end was near. I had the baby monitor on my desk, listening.

The monitor had a setting that blocks out background noise, only registering a difference in the sound. So sometimes it was quiet. But after a few minutes, I realized it'd been too quiet for too long. I adjusted the volume and changed the sensitivity level. Nothing. I turned off the monitor and went upstairs.

I entered the room and found Doris laying still; the labored breathing that had begun earlier that day had subsided. I went to the bed and took her hand. I knew she was gone.

I sat for a few minutes holding her still-warm hand. I put my forehead to her arm and silently cried. I stole those moments for myself before I went downstairs to tell my sister-in-law and before I called Gary to tell him to come home. I whispered that I loved her.

***

Three weeks later, I sat in her armchair, staring at the blue wall. In the same way that I'd transformed the room into my craft room in the days soon after my daughter Sarah left, I'd tried to return the room to the state it was in before Doris came to live with us. The hospital bed was gone, but remnants of her belongings still lingered. Now the closet held Doris' photos and clothes alongside Sarah's stuffed animals and craft supplies I couldn't yet get rid of. I stared at the wall, the one constant element in a room that had witnessed so much change and loss in the past two years.

I knew, then, that a fresh coat of white paint wouldn't erase the memories of the eighteen years Sarah had spent in that room. And it wouldn't have changed my mother-in-law's experiences in the last two months of her life.

That one gesture wouldn't have mattered.

Instead, it was a combination of all of the gestures extended over twenty-eight years that made the difference. The dinners shared. The advice requested. The times I looked the other way when she spoiled her granddaughters. The loyalty to her son and making him happy. Maybe it was okay that I'd left the wall alone. Perhaps I'd done enough.

Jill Wilbur Smith received an M.F.A. in creative writing from Hamline University in St. Paul, Minnesota. Her work has appeared in A Cup of Comfort for Parents of Children with Autism, *in the anthology* Siblings: Our First Macrocosm, *and in the online journal Mothers Always Write. She lives in Minnesota with her husband. She has two grown daughters who are finding their way in life without her daily guidance.*

YOU SPIN ME RIGHT ROUND BABY, RIGHT ROUND
By Alisa Schindler

We were in Pennsylvania for my older son's baseball tournament, and after two days on the sidelines in the dirt and heat, my younger boys had earned a day away from the fields, so I made the mistake of rewarding them with a trip to a nearby amusement park.

Trudging through throngs of exhausted, sweaty parents, I put on the accepting grin of a martyred mom and pushed my 4-year-old in the stroller we thankfully hadn't gotten rid of yet, while my 7-year-old intermittently rode on my back. I would be Super Mom for the day—at least that's what I pretended as I trailed after my boys racing to get in line for the turtle tilt-a-whirl.

Happy to no longer be a mule, I mindlessly watched the ride as we waited for our turn. It resembled those tea cups at every county fair that spin round and round, swirling children into little laughing blurs, only instead of tea cups, this ride had giant turtle shells. I was hesitant to get on the ride. Since reaching the age of 40, spin rides and I are no longer friends, but turtles are notoriously slow creatures, I reasoned, and settled myself in my shell betwixt my two boys.

About fifteen seconds in, with my organs flattened against my back and bile rising in my throat, I realized I'd been tricked by some mad hatter. These were no tea cups! These were turtles on steroids. *Whip! Whip! Whirrrr!* Who would purposely want their head spinning like this without having first enjoyed three margaritas, dancing on a bar, and falling into a bush? Clearly not Julius, my whimpering 4-year-old, who clung to me pitifully, howling like a dying cat.

Around the next turn, breakfast threatening to come back up, I caught a glimpse of my 7-year-old, Michael, his mouth wide open with hysteria, but not the kind Julius and I were experiencing—the excited kind. "Wheeeee!" He screamed and laughed. "Wheeeeee!"

I might've been the one on the verge of throwing up, but he was the real sicko, I thought, as the turtle spun out of control again, pinning me and my thoughts to the shell. As Julius wailed in agony, thoughts of my father flashed in my head. *Would I be happier if he weren't alive?* What? Why would I think that? And why now?

I tried to ponder but who can ponder while spinning at such a high speed. It's actually the opposite of conditions necessary to ponder. *Oh heavens, make this ride stop!* Somewhere in the deep recess of my brain, the song "Whip It" played like a crazy mantra, numbing me until, at last, the turtle took his final turn and died. I mean, the turtle stopped. (I just like to think it died.)

It took all my inner strength to shakily push the safety bar forward. Julius looked almost as shell-shocked as I was, but Michael appeared strangely alert, his eyes a buzz with excitement. "Can we do it again?" He begged. "Please!"

I ignored him, which seemed best since I feared if I opened my mouth, I couldn't be certain what would come out.

***

While the boys wasted money trying to win a twenty-five cent stuffed tiger, I contemplated my ride from hell. *I'm old*, was my first thought. Never would I spin again, except of course, on Tuesday mornings on a stationary bike in the dark with twenty other sweating women. Then there was that *other* random dark thought to deal with, but it was so depressing. *Would I be happier with my father gone?* I mean really? Where did that thought come from? How did my brain make the leap from fun park tilt-a-whirl ride to my troubled father? Was it from his being sick? Constantly out of control? Desperate? Miserable? Even turtles and their slowness were an appropriate connection to my mentally and physically challenged father. Still, there was no denying it was a strange thing to think and a strange place to think it.

Perhaps the thought was a delayed response to the

fact that his number had come up on my cell phone not long before getting on the ride. Simply seeing his number appear on my phone can turn my mood dark quicker than a flick of a light switch. It almost always means trouble. Has he started a fire in his apartment? Did he leave the water running, causing a flood? Has he lost money? Medication? Does he need a doctor? Is he on the ledge wanting to jump, needing a voice to calm him?

As a child, I never consciously realized anything was amiss. Sure, my dad spent a lot of time in bed, and he and my mother fought constantly, but to me, he was playful and funny. He concocted stories at the edge of my bed at night and played extravagant games of hide-and-seek with my cousins, brother, and me, scurrying through a darkened house, hiding in corners, hearts pumping, terrified and exhilarated, listening to his heavy-footed stomps and growls, "I'm gonna get you!"

He bribed us to tickle and massage his back and handed us money on the sly to play video games and buy candy. He was good looking and strong, with Popeye-like muscles and twinkling green eyes. What child would notice or care if he smelled of scotch, worked irregularly, and smoked a lot of funny cigarettes? I sure didn't.

Years passed and my parents divorced. While visiting my father on weekends, red flags snapped like the towels he playfully whipped at us. He lived in squalor, one depressing apartment after another, sleeping on a mattress on the floor with empty liquor bottles scattered about. Still, I was a teenager and didn't live with him. I could ignore it. We went to double features and arcades, and I went back to worrying about myself.

Mental illness is sneaky and difficult to wrap your head around, especially when it comes in a charming package, but unfortunately, as an adult, I couldn't avoid the reality. My father's struggles with addiction, depression, and anxiety overwhelmed him and his health suffered. He blamed a lot of his troubles on a botched back operation that ultimately led to years of chronic pain and pharmaceutical dependence. He lost or gave up his friends, and had never cultivated any significant romantic relationship after he split with my mother. His own father, whom he had little to do with anyway, was gone and his mother, with whom he had a complicated, tumultuous relationship, lived far away in Florida. Which left only me.

Marriage and three children later, the pressures of his troubled, pain-filled life follow me like a shadow every day. There is no escape, not even at a Pennsylvania amusement park. It's now my abnormal-normal, which I sometimes forget other people don't deal with.

I still recall the horrified reaction from a mom when she came to the door to pick up her son, who was playing with my son, at the same time my father's name appeared on my caller ID. I had just been on the phone with him for over an hour and was emotionally exhausted. "Oh it's just my father. He's threatening to kill himself again. I'll call him back," I chirped gaily. The woman took her child and backed slowly away. I don't think our sons ever "played" again, but at least she didn't call the cops.

While waving to the boys now on the merry-go-round, I listened to my father's message. Just watching the horses go round was making me nauseous, but sadly, my father's message made me dizzier still.

"Lis, uh LIS, yeah hi. Hi! I'm having some problems. Shit. Why do I do this? Uh, right, so um. Jaylee didn't show again. I'm so stupid. Everything's a mess. I'm confused. Can you call me? Yeah, call me. Ok. Sorry. *Sorry*! Ok. I don't know what's going on. I'll try you at home again. Where are you? Are you not talking to me? Why do I screw everything up? Sorry. sorry. Bye . . ." Phone clanking, banging, falling. A muffled, "Ow" before the click and then silence.

Sigh. Really? I'd spoken with him the day before and told him I was away with the family and probably wouldn't speak with him for a couple of days. He had his home health aide, who apparently didn't show up that day, although it wouldn't be surprising if he'd told her not to come or had kicked her out. Anything was possible.

I didn't want to deal with one of his disasters now. In

fact, I *couldn't* deal with one. I had two children and was at an amusement park in another state. Being distracted was not an option. He'd have to wait.

***

Michael and Julius bounded up to me, fresh from their steeds and demanded to have their faces painted. While a face full of paint in ninety-degree heat didn't sound appealing to me, I obliged. I was still pretending to be Super Mom, and I hoped they were buying it as much as I was paying for it. Cotton candy? No problem. Face painting? Of course. Ice cream? Why not! Twenty dollars to win an ugly stuffed fish? Hell yeah! Sky's the limit here in Super Mommy Town.

"Happy?" I asked my boys, now transformed to Spiderman Michael and Julius the Puppy.

Julius the Puppy wagged his tail. Michael, the dark superhero said, "Can we go now?"

Having survived the day reasonably unscathed—even, dare I say, successfully—I automatically agreed, thrilled to not press my luck any further.

Back in the car with my two boys safe, buckled in and ready to nod off, I debated whether to call my father back and provide a Band-Aid to his unfixable problems. I'd never set foot on a tilt-a-whirl again; yet every day I ride my father's never-ending emotional roller coaster.

Obligation and responsibility are part of who I am.

I can't walk away. I can only do my best for him, for myself, and for my family. Generally they are at odds with each other, but would I be happier if he were gone from my life? The answer is no. Even with the heavy burden I help him carry, when I look in the mirror his green eyes look back.

Still, it would be nice to take a long vacation from having a father with unsolvable problems and from being a daughter whose head is constantly spinning.

Sighing, I dial his number.

Alisa Schindler is the mom of three boys and wife to Mr. Baseball. She schlepps children, burns cupcakes, and writes essays that have been featured online at the New York Times; Washington Post; *Kveller; Brain, Child;* Woman's Day; Parents; *and* Good Housekeeping, *among others. She is a 2016 Voices of the Year and occasionally blogs at icescreammama.com. Her not at all depressing fiction novels,* Secrets of the Suburbs *and* Murder Across the Street, *are available on Amazon.*

TOMORROW NEVER COMES
By Georgia A. Hubley

I was startled awake when the phone rang on the nightstand by my bed. Through blurry eyes, I squinted at the illuminated 4:00 a.m. in green numerals on the alarm clock and grappled for the phone.

I was surprised to hear Mom's voice at the other end of the phone, and that she'd forgotten there was a three-hour time difference between the east coast and the west coast. I assumed she was calling about my upcoming visit, but that was not the case.

"Hon, what time is it, seven o'clock a.m. or seven o'clock p.m.?" she asked after I'd groggily answered the phone.

Remembering how much she enjoyed morning TV, I was certain I knew how to show her what time it was.

"Mom, are you watching your favorite TV weatherman, Al Roker, on the *Today Show*?" I asked.

Exasperated, she groaned loudly, "No, I don't have time to watch TV. I need to take my pills. It's dark outside and I can't tell if it's morning or nighttime."

"Mom, it's seven o'clock a.m. where you are," I said.

There was no immediate reply, but I could hear her stirring about and mumbling about being late in taking her pills.

"Mom, are you there?" I yelled, hoping she'd hear me and return to the phone.

A minute later she picked up the phone and announced, "I'm back! I just took my pills. I'm hanging up now. Hon, I'll be seeing you soon."

I was unable to return to sleep. I felt helpless being thousands of miles away.

In a week's time, Mom's forgetfulness worsened. She forgot a pan cooking on the stove and the fire department was called to her rescue. Then she over-medicated herself by taking double the dosage of her heart medication and was rushed to the hospital. I was so grateful my brother and family didn't live far away.

***

Several weeks later, Mom was diagnosed with Alzheimer's disease. Sadly, my fun-loving mom, once an independent woman and widow of fifteen years, was no longer capable of caring for herself or her affairs. Heart-wrenching as it was, there was no other choice but to have her cared for at a convalescent facility.

During my flight to the east coast, my thoughts drifted back to how Mom and I used to laugh when she'd say, "I'm having a senior moment," every time she forgot the name of a person, place, or thing. After all, her friends forgot things. I know that neither of us thought that one day she'd be diagnosed with Alzheimer's disease.

When I arrived at the facility to visit Mom, I was told she was waiting for me on their enclosed patio. As I approached, I hoped she'd see me, smile, and wave hello. But there was no recognition.

I leaned down, gave Mom a hug, and announced my arrival. She appeared confused but motioned for me to sit down beside her and said, "You can visit with me until my daughter arrives."

I wanted to bolt from the room, but I didn't. Instead, I sat down next to her and held her hand. She smiled and asked, "What is your name?"

"My name is Georgia," I replied.

Although I was devastated, I pretended it didn't matter. Quickly, I realized her attention span was almost nonexistent and that a conversation between us was impossible. However, I talked to her anyway, sharing my precious memories—many the same ones that eluded her.

As I contemplated what to say next, a faint rumble of thunder startled me. I noticed raindrops on the windowpanes. I watched lightning zigzag across the sky. Suddenly, there was a deafening crash of thunder that made me flinch. I squeezed Mom's hand too hard, but she didn't seem to mind.

"When I was a little girl my house was struck by lightning," I said.

Mom seemed attentive, so I felt compelled to share a chapter from the story of our lives she'd forgotten:

"Mom, one summer evening when I was 9 and my brother 7, thunder clamored and lightning crackled overhead drowning out your words as you read the Sunday comics to us. The three of us snuggled close in Dad's favorite brown overstuffed chair, while we waited for the storm to subside.

"Suddenly, a bolt of lightning struck the wall behind us, its force so intense we were thrown from the overstuffed chair. The room was in total darkness. Stunned by the sudden jolt, I wondered why I was sprawled on the floor. Lightning flashed, and to my surprise there was a gaping hole in the wall, with electrical sparks flying about the room and the taste and smell of burned sulphur in the air. I was too terrified to scream or cry.

"Unrelenting flashes of lightning made it possible to catch a glimpse of my brother crawling toward you as you lay motionless on the floor several feet away.

"As I groped through the debris to join you, Dad, who'd been working in the barn, charged through the front door carrying a lantern, 'Are you all okay?' he asked. 'I heard an explosion.'

"'Something's wrong with Mom,' I whimpered.

"We watched Dad tend to you. Repeatedly, he called out your name, 'Annie, Annie, Annie. Please wake up.'

"I was so relieved when you finally spoke, my head hurt. What happened? Why are we on the floor?' you asked.

"'Take it easy, you were knocked out cold for a while,' Dad said.

"Thankfully, neighbors came to our aid and helped Dad board up the huge hole in the wall, and treated the small gash on the side of your head. None of us could sleep a wink, as the storm raged on through the night.

"Early the next morning, the storm moved on and patches of blue sky appeared overhead. It was soon discovered that lightning had struck a telephone pole and followed the phone line that led into our house, which caused the wall phone to explode. A large battery from inside the phone had hit your head and caused you to lose consciousness. Fortunately, you weren't seriously injured and our house wasn't engulfed in flames . . ."

I paused . . . then ended the story, "And that's why I'm afraid of thunderstorms."

Mom grinned and patted my hand, "Hon, I don't like thunderstorms either."

I gave her a hug, kissed her cheek, and prepared to leave. "Mom, I love you," I said. "I'll see you tomorrow."

A puzzled expression crossed Mom's face, "But tomorrow never comes," she said.

***

The doctors and the nurses refer to Mom as "pleasantly confused." Even though she doesn't recognize anyone and her memories are lost, she's never lost her sweet disposition. From her bedroom window, she admires the beautiful flowers in the facility's gardens, and she giggles while watching squirrels scamper across the lawn or up the trees. She enjoys sitting on the patio and watching everyone who enters the facility. She no longer wears a watch. She seems content never having to worry about what time it is.

Mom's memory banks are empty and mine are overflowing. I continue telling her stories and she listens.

Georgia A. Hubley grew up on a seventy-acre farm without the modern conveniences of indoor plumbing, electricity, or a telephone. Therefore, she became an avid reader and knew one day she'd become a writer. She retired after twenty years from financial management in Silicon Valley to write full-time. Her short stories and essays appear in various anthologies and periodicals. After two sons were launched into adulthood and the nest was empty, Georgia and her husband relocated to the Nevada desert.

TEN YEARS
By Christine Carter

"I figure I've got about ten years left."

My father said these words to me during one of our visits. His comment seemed to come out of nowhere, somehow landing in the midst of our casual conversation. I glanced toward the sky as my chest trapped my breath, unable to fully process my father's words, grasping at this undeniable and relentless truth he claimed. I can't remember what we were discussing or what we were doing, but his prophetic words continue to echo through my thoughts to this day.

Ten years? Ten? Ten years . . . Ten. Years.

I hadn't thought of his life limited, his life ending, his life anything but vital and ongoing. I didn't need to, because my father had always been the pillar of great health in every single way. His stature commanded confidence; his unyielding strength exuded stamina and success. I had no reason to apply life's mortality to a man who never faltered or failed and surely never appeared fragile or frayed. There was no time limit, no concern for embracing what's left of life, never a need to count the years, the days, the moments.

Ten years . . .

Those words still can't find a place to settle in my heart. They bounce through my thoughts, tear through my mind, and break open a part of me that whispers, *his time is limited*, triggering regrets and questions in rapid speed.

Why didn't I visit more or call more through the years . . . and why don't I now?

He may never see my kids get married. He won't be there to watch them grow into adults and have children of their own. He rarely sees them now: neither my daughter racing in the water, nor my son dominating on the soccer field. He's missed so many triumphant moments in their short lives already. We've both already missed so much.

I wonder if he feels the same. I wonder if he thinks of these things. I wonder if he, too, allows regret to slip into the folds of his heart, wanting to make it all different than what is has been, what it is, what it will be.

The reality is that things won't change. Our fleeting time together doesn't exist in the day-to-day. We live too far away from each other to dive into the depths of those significant details, so we touch base briefly through phone calls and e-mails. I'm already mourning his absence and this loss of time we keep missing.

Ten years . . .

I panic at times, devastated at the idea of my father's life ending. I can't allow this panic to penetrate any deeper or I'll be paralyzed at the enormity of its truth. Who really knows how many years anyone has left? But aging seems to slowly ignite that immanent question within us all.

I often string a thousand wishes together of all those things we should've done and all those things we cannot change. I also reflect on those days when we lived our finest moments, both together and apart. Major life changes and transitions that punctuate our years are strong pillars in the groundwork of who I am. There have been times my dad showed up when I needed him most, revealing his care and concern during my heartbreaks and hard times. I'll always treasure such tender moments I felt his love and devotion so deeply. Those vivid memories are sewn into my heart and threaded through all the facets of who I am.

***

In the past few years, my father and I have grown more connected in ways I wished we had when I was younger. Perhaps life has stripped some of his hardened exterior and supernatural drive that used to intimidate me. Maybe I've grown enough to see the father he's always been, as my vision cleared with maturity. With the barriers more faint, I now notice softening layers of emotion rise up from within his increasingly subdued nature. I embrace his new sensitivities in each phone conversation, e-mail update, and any visit we have. My dad will always be a man of integrity, honesty, and commitment. Through my forty-nine years, he's never stopped being consistent and, more importantly, he's always been a steady force of influence in my life.

We've endured challenges along the way, as all families do. There have been bouts of conflicts and trials that have left brokenness in their wake. Life does that. It splatters futile fragments all over the walls of our fragile existence, leaving us to clean up the mess. Despite those painful circumstances, my dad has always tried to be present during the clean up. His love has been a stabilizing anchor in some pretty fierce storms I've managed to survive.

I wonder if he knows that.

Ten years . . .

I've spent most of my life desperately craving his attention, his affirmation, his assurance while his unfaltering views and perspectives often paved a path my feet couldn't find. Despite the dividing intersections we approached, he never stopped believing in me as I set out to place my own sometimes wavering footing on freshly built ground. My father's dream for my success looked differently than my own, and yet, he'd prove over and over again that wherever my feet would land, he'd have confidence in who I am and the direction I dreamed to go.

I'm an "Epkins" through and through, and I can only hope to live the legacy my father and his father birthed through hard work, intention, and an impeccably positive perspective. I'll never stop building on the values and principles that radiate from his life, as I continue to instill the same standards in my own children. Now in this more intimate season he and I have entered, I bask in the grace he pours onto me and the acceptance he humbly offers in everything I do, believe, or voice. His praise and encouragement lift me to a place of courage and inspiration. I soak in this sweetness as it saturates my soul.

Even grown adults need their parent's love.

Ten years . . .

***

My dad is nearing 80 years old. Ten years seem magical, almost lavish. He's proven mind-over-matter time and time again, having rarely ever been sick, and I've yet to see the man tired. He doesn't stop going and doing and achieving and working and embracing every single day to its fullest. He's witnessed age take down many of his beloved friends and colleagues. I wonder how often he summons his mind as weaponry against these odds. He's well aware of his timeline, for mind can never defeat death.

Oh God, how I wish it could.

His age is showing little by little in his appearance and his stature. I struggle to write those words, because that means they're documented as evidence my dad's life is nearing the end.

Time is running out, speeding toward the finish line, and there's nothing we can do about it. I wonder what my dad wishes for, worries about, or dreams during these days. I can't comprehend the intensity of it all, nor do I want to. Not now, not ever. But I have no choice. None of us do.

In my silent moments, I think of him and want to change time and change me. I want to spend every moment I possibly can with him, and yet I know that won't happen, because raising a family hundreds of miles away requires my attention and devotion, leaving little room for more than a few visits every now and then. A painful yet accurate excuse. One I swallow down hard and challenge myself to rearrange so I can cling to the man who's had the greatest impact on my life and embrace the time I still have with him.

Ten years . . . they're going by so fast.

Chris Carter is a stay-at-home mom of two amazing kids. Her 10-year-old son and 13-year-old daughter keep her pretty darn busy, along with running a weekly youth ministry and women's ministry out of her home. Five years into motherhood, she quit her career to focus solely on caring for her daughter's growing medical needs. Once her daughter's health was restored, Chris decided to pursue her lifetime love of writing. She created TheMomCafe.com with a mission to encourage women through her humor, inspiration, and faith. Her work can also be seen on HuffingtonPost, ScaryMommy, Mamapedia, ForEveryMom, HerViewFromHome, MomBabble and more.

MOVING NANA IN
By Ambrosia Brody

"Will you be our full-time babysitter?" my husband, Alex, and I asked my mom over speakerphone two years ago after she told us she'd been laid off.

The timing was perfect since I was pregnant with our first daughter.

"Of course," she said, "but how will that work? Will I drive to Orange County every morning?"

"We'd like to move you from Los Angeles to be closer to us," Alex explained.

"Oh, really?" she asked, falling silent.

"Mom, it's okay if you don't want to do it," I said.

"No, it's fine. If it wasn't I'd tell you," she said. "I think I'll like it."

***

Living in a multigenerational household is not uncommon for our family. My mom and I lived in my grandmother's house in East Los Angeles for the first eight years of my life, the same three-bedroom house where my grandma raised nine children.

We had a room to ourselves where we shared a large four-post bed and chest of drawers. My mom carved out a corner of the room for my things: a small table where I played with Play-Doh and kept my pet fish Rainbow.

That's where our personal space ended.

Outside our room, the rest of the house was alive with movement. Family members always seemed to be around gathering at the house for a bowl of *menudo* or stopping by to see Grandma, often dropping off one of my cousins for Grandma to babysit.

My days were filled with building forts underneath the living room table with cousins, walking down to Ford Boulevard for *pan dulce*, or tagging along with Grandma and her sister, Tia Lala, to the salon where they'd get their hair cut and styled. On hot summer days, when Popsicles weren't enough to keep us kids cool, Grandma would allow us to strip down to our underwear, and she would wet us with the hose in the front yard.

At night, I'd sneak into Grandma's room because I knew she'd talk my mom into allowing me to stay up a little longer, snuggling with her under the heavy comforter and watching novellas together.

For my mom, living with her parents meant home-cooked meals, saving on childcare, and knowing that her mom and sisters were always there to help. And Grandma was always around, only leaving the house when one of her children picked her up for the day. Even on those evenings when my mom came home late from work, Grandma waited up, warming a plate of food and sitting with her, catching up on the day.

"*Su hija le gusta un chico*," she whispered one evening as my mom washed the dishes.

"What? How do you know she likes a boy?" my mom asked.

"*Fue en ese cuaderno en la mesa*," she said, alerting my mom of the journal I kept.

Privacy and silence were two things you could never find at Grandma's—even at night the sounds of Grandma's TV, firecrackers, and ranchero music from a neighbor's house drowned out the silence.

***

My mom's move to Orange County—or the OC, as it's often called—signified a new beginning for both of us: hers as a grandma and mine as a new mom.

Every morning, my mom would drive the ten-minute route from her apartment to our house to care for our first born, Brynna, while Alex and I were at work.

She and Brynna quickly found their groove: visiting the library, attending Gymboree, and when Brynna was older, working on her Spanish and numbers.

It took me a little longer to navigate the terrain of being a new mom with my mom as my daughter's nanny. That first year I felt the stress of being her main source of income, feeling guilty that we couldn't pay her more to compensate for all that we asked of her. Not only was she working long hours caring for Brynna, but she had relocated, moving away from her sisters in L.A., whom she visited on a weekly basis.

I worried she was lonely on the weekends since she couldn't see her sisters as often, and I was too preoccupied with my own little family to take her to a movie or the mall. I pestered her to go to the doctor when she'd get sick and worried I wasn't able to give her a much-needed vacation.

The stress of being my mom's employer, daughter, health monitor, and host began to weigh on my shoulders.

"Don't worry about me, *Mija*," she'd say whenever I'd tell her how guilty I felt that she was so far from her sisters, or that I couldn't take the time off to allow her to spend a few weeks in New York with her sister. "It's fine," she'd say. "If it wasn't, I'd tell you."

When we found out I was pregnant with our second child, Alex and I agreed it made sense to move her in with us.

"She basically lives with us already, and she helps out a lot," Alex reminded me during one of our do-we-move-mom-in discussions.

"But what if, by the time we no longer need her help, she can't move out?" I asked. "Like does this mean she'll always live with us?"

"I don't know," he said. "But at least you won't have

to worry about her being alone."

***

When I was in high school, I watched as my mom and *tias* cared for Grandma when her health deteriorated. They moved her into our old room, replacing our four-post bed with a hospital bed; they learned to feed her through a feeding tube, popping open the Ensure tab, dispensing the strawberry or vanilla liquid into the tube. They propped her up on pillows, bathed her, changed her clothes, combed her hair, and massaged her feet, arms, and hands.

They made sure she was never alone, rearranging their schedules to be with her.

Her daughters were with her when she passed away, rubbing her legs and hands, telling her it was okay to go, that they would be okay; they had each other.

***

Brynna loves having her Nana in the house. She spends time with her each night before bedtime. Sometimes they watch TV together; other times they have a tickle session resulting in Brynna's laughter floating down the stairs, filling every empty space of the house with the sweet sound of happiness.

"Oh, I'm going to Nana's room just for a little bit," she'll announce when I tell her it's almost time for bed.

"Mom, just let me know if you need a break. I know

you've been with the girls all day," I yell from the bottom of the stairs as Brynna runs upstairs.

"It's fine. If it wasn't, I'd tell you," she calls back.

My daughter loves my mom's room where she builds forts out of pillows and sorts through her Nana's jewelry playing dress-up.

The weight of being everything to my mom is heavy at times, but for the most part, her living with us has alleviated many of my fears. We've fallen into a routine, and she makes plans on the weekends to have her own time. Somehow, this arrangement is working for us—for now.

"Bedtime," I tell my youngest daughter as I hand her off to my mom so I can get Brynna to bed.

"Kiss and hug goodnight," Brynna says, leaning into my mom for a kiss.

"Goodnight, *Corazon*," my mom calls after us as we walk to Brynna's room.

"Did you have a good day with Nana?" I ask while tucking her into bed.

"I sure did," she whispers. "Does Nana live in my home?" she asks.

"She sure does," I whisper back.

"I like that," she says.

"Yeah, me too," I say, before kissing her goodnight.

Ambrosia Brody is a full-time editor, journalist, and mother to two spirited daughters. She lives in Southern California in a beach city but hates the sand; she enjoys people watching but hates small talk. She started to blog at randomaspectsofmylife.blogspot.com when she realized everything she knew about parenting was wrong.

AT THE BRIDGE OF GODS
By R. Todd Fredrickson

"That sure is a long train."

I looked over at my 81-year-old father who was sitting shotgun in my '70 C10 pickup. He was snapping a yellowed thumbnail under the metal clip of the seat belt.

"Leave that alone," I said, pushing his hand away. "I don't want it coming unlatched and then you go face first into the dashboard if I have to brake hard."

"That train sure is long," he said, as if I didn't hear him the first time.

"It's two trains," I said. "The first one was going west and this one is going east."

He rolled his window down and watched the train's engine move beyond the bend. Every other car had a flatbed that was empty; the others were the box and cage type laced with graffiti.

"Double tracks in the middle of a town this size," he said. "It doesn't make any sense. What if an ambulance is trying to cross the tracks?"

"I know," I said. "I've never understood it myself. But what do we little mushrooms know anyway, huh?"

Dad snorted and then smiled. "Politicians."

"Yup."

The last train had an engine at the end. It looked like it was pushing the line rather than being pulled. The bar raised and we moved slowly across the tracks. I'm aware that our bodies dance the same movement, our heads bob side to side, and then our butts slide forward on the seat. We both stiffen our legs to push our hips back.

His driver's license still says his hair is white, but it's more like spent charcoal in the barbeque. Mine says red, but it had always been more orange than red. Now, when I see my hair clippings in my lap at the barber shop, I only see the hair of an old guy. Other than the buzz-cut hair style, my dad and I don't look so much alike.

Mom always said I took after her dad, same blue eyes and same temperament at least. I don't know, maybe I'm a little of both of them.

"How are you feeling?" I said.

"I think I have to go to the bathroom."

"What do you mean 'you think' you have to go?" I said.

"I can wait until we get there; I'm okay."

I look at him for signs of distress or pain but only see contentment. His hands are in his lap, long, boney fingers laced between knuckles that've always reminded me of the back of the ball-peen hammer that hung on the wall in the garage next to jars of screws, bolts, and nails for as long as I can remember. Those same hands suffered the elements of the Korean War, held the soft hands of his 19-year-old wife, carried me into the North Cascades to Alpine Lakes, and touched the cheek of my mother, his wife, when she took her last breath.

"It's a long drive into Oregon, Dad," I said. "We'll make a stop once we get through Seattle. Grab a coffee and something sweet."

"The final supper, huh?" he said.

"It's never too late to change your mind," I said, trying to gauge his comment.

"No, it's time, Son."

***

Three months ago, Dad called me and asked that I stop by for a visit. He still lived in the house he and Mom had bought in the early sixties and went on to raise my sister Jolene and me in. The fields where my sister and I acted out scenes from *The Lone Ranger* have since become the sites of new home developments, houses crammed together so close there was no room for a backyard barbecue. Along with the dense housing came increased traffic and noise. Mom wanted to move, but Dad wouldn't hear it.

"I'm not going to let those noisy so-n-so's push me out of the neighborhood I've invested in all my life!" he'd say before slamming the screen door on his way out.

When the county gave the okay for commercial flights out of a major airline assembly plant, the routes flew over the house. Most of them were high enough that the noise was minimal, but some came in lower and rattled the plates in the cupboard. Mom called me at work on more than one occasion to tell me that Dad was in the backyard flipping the bird at the airplanes again.

"I'm worried," she said. "His stubbornness is going to be the end of him."

"He's just expressing himself, Mom," I'd say. "Don't put too much thought into it."

Later that spring, I showed up to cut their grass; as I was putting away the mower, I spotted a big red "number one" foam hand from high school tucked behind a box of Christmas ornaments. I took it down and tried it on. It still fit my hand like a clown glove. I cut the finger off and quickly glued it back on over the middle knuckle. Mom and Dad were in the living room watching the news when I entered with it.

"Look Dad, those airplanes will be able to see your finger now!" I said, laughing hard. He glanced at the giant foam middle finger and then back at me, assessing whether I was making fun of him.

"Put it on the patio, and I'll give it a try next time," he said, turning back to the TV.

He never got a chance to use it. Mom had tossed it into the trash the day the garbage truck came around. She denied doing so, but I saw the defiant spark of truth in her eyes. I let it go after that.

A year to that date, Mom passed away in her sleep. Natural causes, they said. Dad's soul was bruised from the loss, and he never returned to the person he was when he'd been with the love of his life. He became quiet and uninterested in holding a conversation aside from basic questions about my family or job. When he called me at work after a few weeks of not answering my calls to ask me to stop by his house, I took it as a sign of recovery from depression. But when he opened the door, the first thing I noticed were the whites of his eyes, which were not white at all, but instead, the color of a coffee stain on the tablecloth.

"Dad, what did you do to your eyes?"

"How the hell should I know!" he said, walking away. "Why do you think I called you?"

I walked in and closed the door behind me. The kitchen was a mess, and I doubted he had washed dishes in a week.

"Do they hurt?"

"My eyes?" he said. "No, they feel funny, heavy, but they don't hurt."

I immediately took him to the Valley Clinic in town. The young assistant asked if he'd ever had hepatitis. Dad started yelling at her about how he'd spent two years in Korea and never once got dysentery or chlamydia, let alone hepatitis. I felt bad for the nurse who took the brunt of his temper. She handled it like a pro, though, patting his hand and thanking him for his service.

"Have you experienced any back pain?" she said.

"Nothing more than an old man experiences when his frame is breaking down."

"How about your diet?" she said. "Are you eating well?"

"I'm by myself now so I might not be eating like I did when my wife was around."

"What did you have for breakfast today?"

"A cup of coffee and a piece of toast," he said, crossing his arms across his chest.

"Dad, you're eating like a bird!"

He looked at me and didn't say anything, but it was clear he wanted me to mind my own business.

"How about your bowel movements?" she continued.

"What about them?" he said, his cheeks flushed.

"Are they normal?"

"I don't know. What's normal?"

"Well, everyone has their own schedule, so you know what's normal for you."

He looked over at me and then back to her. His hands were in his lap, and he was picking at the yellow thumbnail.

"I suppose the schedule is a little off," he said. "And the color is off also."

"The color of the bowel movements?" she asked.

"I thought that's what we were talking about?"

"Have you noticed blood in your stool?"

"No blood," he said. "It's just a lighter color. Like the clay dirt under the topsoil in the garden."

"Have you lost any weight?"

"I don't know about that," he said, pulling at his belt.

He was referred to a specialist in Everett, and, after a battery of tests over several days, they diagnosed him with pancreatic cancer.

***

He first hinted at the idea of taking things into his own hands after the last visit to the oncology surgeon, who had told him his cancer was aggressive and advanced. The best the doctor could do was minimize or delay the discomfort Dad felt.

We were sitting in my car in his driveway after the appointment when Dad said, "I don't see the point."

"What do you mean?"

"I mean I have three months, maybe four, before my body gives up the ghost."

He was right, of course, it wasn't easy hearing him admit it, but he seemed resigned to that reality. That didn't make it any easier to hear, however.

"If I had a gun, I'd just end it on my own." he said.

"Now *that's* ridiculous!"

"Sure, I know," he said. "I let my life insurance policy expire after your mother passed. I figured I was too old for it anyway. Us old folks get charged maximum rates, because they know we aren't going to pay into it much longer."

He was looking down at his feet, his hands were on his thighs, and the thumbs were rubbing the inside of his knees.

"Funny," he said. "My knees really ache. I hadn't noticed it before the doctor suggested joint pain."

"I don't give a rip about any life insurance or estate, Dad!"

"You and your sister are good that way," he said. "Your mother did a great job."

"You both did."

"It would be too messy anyway," he said.

"What's that?"

"You know—if I shot myself or some other thing."

I didn't know what to say. We were talking about him taking his own life to end the inevitable. It was like taking too big of a bite of a sandwich: it's going to be a while before it's processed enough to swallow.

"Come on, let's go in," I said and got out of the car.

I didn't look back to see if he was following, but when I was on the porch pulling the key, I heard the car door shut. I walked through the house and into the kitchen to put on some coffee. He was still using the same stove top percolator he and mom bought right after they were married. Like a lot of things in the house, he didn't see a point replacing it since it still served its purpose. He'd still be using a rotary phone if the phone company hadn't told him he couldn't use it anymore because it slowed down the lines. It sounded kind of fishy to me, but I bought them a push-button cordless phone anyway. Mom liked the change, being able to sit out on the porch and talk with her sister in Idaho, rather than being stuck at the wall phone.

"I think Oregon got it right," Dad said, as I was pouring coffee into a mug that read, "Proud member of the Grumpy Old Man Club."

"What's that?"

"The Death with Dignity bill those liberals down there passed a few years back."

Dad had a habit of classifying people based on their politics and his personal beliefs. He was more liberal than he'd admit. Veterans from his generation leaned to one party, because they thought it was a respectful thing to do for the current veterans. I'd pointed out that the elected officials he was voting for, who were always talking war and yelling at someone, were also trying to balance the budget by increasing his costs as a retiree, while sending his tax dollar to other countries for questionable reasons. After that speech, he paid more attention to the resume than a party affiliation.

We sat at the kitchen table with our coffee. Neither one of us said anything for a moment. I wasn't sure if he was just talking nonsense or being serious.

"We need to tell your sister," he finally said.

"Would you like me to or do you want to?"

"It might be easier if you did," he said. "She'll come over when she's ready."

I waited a day to tell Jolene so I could let my mind-chatter settle a little and set my thoughts straight. I could hear her crying on the other end, and then she said she was going over to see him.

Dad had given me his word he wouldn't do anything drastic, suggesting he was just kidding, but I could tell that wasn't the whole truth. When I got home, I looked up the Oregon bill he'd mentioned. The person had to be a resident of the state of Oregon. Strike one. And they had to have the written permission from the doctor that would provide the prescription. Strike two.

That night Jolene called. She was still at Dad's house. I could hear his TV in the background. He was a creature of habit.

"This is just wrong," she said.

"I would agree," I said, assuming she was talking about his health and not his affliction with the TV.

"I can't believe there isn't anything they can do for

him. I mean really, he doesn't even look sick!"

"I know," I said. "Other than his eyes."

"He wants to move to Oregon," I said, hoping to ease into the topic.

"He told me."

"And?"

There was a long pause. She was crying. I wanted to also but was afraid I wouldn't be able to stop.

"From what I read, the last month or so will be miserable for him, even in hospice," she said.

"Agreed then?" I said, holding my breath to delay the leaking dam.

"Yes."

We both hung up. I dropped to the floor and bawled like a child.

***

It took three weeks to get Dad's doctor to provide a referral to an Oregon doctor who was familiar with the Death with Dignity Act. I suspect they discussed ethical and professional concerns, but ultimately Dad received the call confirming the date for the first interview. Jolene found him an assisted living home in Hood River, and the move to Oregon happened quickly. The only person who knew of his request, other than Jolene and me, was his doctor.

Just short of two months into his stay, his health

started to decline. He didn't want to get out of bed and, when he would, he required a walker to maneuver around.

He wanted to see his house before it was sold, and he asked that everything happen at a location with a view of Washington, the state where he'd lived his entire life other than twenty-four months in Korea. Jolene found a place that allowed for privacy and was only a short distance from his new assisted-living home.

When I went to pick him up so we could drive back up to Monroe to see his house one last time, he looked frail and gaunt. His breathing was raspy, and he took small steps towards my truck. When I reached the passenger side, I opened the door and started to help him in.

"What are you doing?" he snapped.

"Helping you."

He waved me on. "Throw that damn walker in the back. I can get myself in, thank you."

I loaded the walker and stood by, watching him pull himself in. He struggled a bit, but managed to get in. He fumbled with the seat belt and eventually let me help him with it. When I got in, I looked over at him. He was staring out the window, breathing hard.

"You okay?" I said.

When he looked at me, I saw fear in his eyes. I've never known him to scare easily. Maybe he was simply scared of being afraid.

"Sure, I'm just trying to catch my breath."

I wondered if it was too soon, if he might have more time than we thought. But how close could he get to the end and still be lucid enough to make a rational decision? The state law required that the patient make the end-of-life decision and final act of taking the prescription.

We drove up north and around the old neighborhood. We couldn't get inside the house because Dad had left his keys in his room, and Jolene had my set from when she worked with the agent.

"Let's go," he said.

Once back on the freeway headed to Oregon, I asked him if he was in any pain. There was a long pause between my asking him and his response.

"I remember when you were a little sprout," he said, looking out the side window. "Five, maybe six. You and your sister were helping me feed and water the chickens. Your sister insisted on checking for the eggs first, and so I told her to go ahead and put them in the bucket after we filled the feed bin. You wanted to check them also, and she didn't like that idea, so she pushed you backwards out the door. You fell hard. I heard your noggin bounce off the step. What a terrible sound that was. I pushed her out of the way and leaned out thinking you had split your head open. I pulled you onto my lap and asked you if you were okay, if you were in any pain. You were crying so hard you were gasping for air."

He looked over at me as if he were looking for the same toddler he was talking about.

"It just took the wind out of you and left a nice knot on your head for a while, but boy, nothing could match the pain I felt for you, so helpless, you know."

"Yup, I remember that one," I said, rubbing the spot behind my ear. "I think she was sorry the moment she did it."

"You were pals after that, for sure."

Neither of us spoke as we wound through Seattle and then passed the Lewis-McCord military base, getting closer to the state line, caught up in our own memories from the deep family well. Finally we crossed the Columbia River and headed east down I-84.

"Jolene has the paperwork for you to sign. The only other person who will be there is the notary, but he's going to leave after he stamps his signature," I said.

"Were you able to find a spot with the view I asked for?"

"Yes, I think you'll appreciate it."

A sign on Dad's side of the road read, "Bridge of Gods Next Right."

"There it is." I said.

"Good," Dad said, poking a finger into the pocket where the pills were, looking at the sign and then off toward the river where you could see the bridge span across the Columbia River into Washington State.

"I've missed your mother the last few months more than ever before," he said.

"We all have."

"I know, but it's been strong, this feeling. I think she's been hanging around waiting for me."

"That's a nice thought."

"Still not a believer, huh?"

"I have hope, Dad. It's a nice idea, but that's as far as I can take it at the moment."

He nodded. "I understand."

We pulled into the parking lot and then drove toward the west side where a trail head began. Most of the vehicles parked on the opposite side, because it was closer to walk into town. We parked next to Jolene who was looking over at us with moist, puffy eyes. She waved at Dad, who returned the greeting, smiling back at her and then looking over at me.

"I love you, Dad," I said.

"I love you too, Son. Carry on."

Todd Fredrickson, and his wife, Wendy, live in Monroe Washington, where they enjoy hiking in the Cascades and getting lost in a good book. Todd has published two books, Brothers of the Sun and Moon, *and* A Short Five.

CATCHING UP
By Amy Halzel Willis

The birthday card featured a photo of two little girls, around age 7, dressed in white sundresses and hats and galloping across a field of wildflowers. The caption read, "We shared our childhood together . . ."

Nope, that's not the one, I thought, as I placed the card back on the pharmacy display shelf. While the photo was sweet, the message didn't resonate for me. My sister, Lois, is eleven years older than I am, so we never pranced around in frilly dresses together. By the time I was 7 years old, Lois was leaving our home for college.

My other sister, Cindy, is just two years younger than Lois. She and Lois *did* grow up together, whispering secrets in the bedroom they shared.

Like choosing a birthday card, living life with sisters who are always far ahead of me can be awkward. Whatever stage of life I'm in, not only have they "been there and done that," but they did it a long time ago. When I was in high school and college, they were married and having children. When I was planning my wedding, they were planning their kids' Bar Mitzvah parties.

But despite its peculiarities, being the youngest by a decade has its perks. My sisters and their childhood

friends remember their excitement when I was born, and they still revere me as "the baby." Even better, my grown nieces and nephews affectionately dubbed me "the cool aunt," due, I believe, to my relative youthfulness.

Perhaps most importantly, it can be comforting to have siblings who, with years of experience, offer good advice and counsel. When my husband and I were choosing our first apartment, Lois encouraged me to go with a large unit that Ken liked, but was clearly dated with shag carpet and flowered wallpaper. As much as I loved the spacious floor plan, I couldn't get past the old-lady vibe of the place.

Lois came with me to take a second look. "Once you hang your prints on the walls, it will look trendy," she explained, nodding her head with the conviction of a seasoned decorator.

Sure enough, it did.

When our daughter was born a few years later, I was a sleepless wreck of postpartum hormones and sweatpants. Anxious and a bit terrified of what I was getting myself into, I summoned my sisters in a panic.

Cindy came to the rescue, arriving at my home with a large bag of hand-me-down onesies and receiving blankets. She entertained Juliana by cooing with her, nose-to-nose, while I wolfed down a sandwich between diaper changes and general fretting.

"She's perfect," Cindy assured me, drawing upon her

wealth of maternal wisdom.

Indeed, she was.

***

But the familiar and happy way I'd always thought of myself—as the mega-youngest sister—began to change shortly after I had my second child. As I was deep in the throes of mothering young children, our aging parents both developed health issues. It started slowly at first. Our mother began to have episodes of fever that required hospital stays and blood transfusions. Our father became forgetful and was acting strangely on occasion.

While trying to keep a positive attitude, my sisters and I grew concerned as our parents became increasingly dependent on us to coordinate their medical appointments, help them fill out forms, and shop for them. Even when they were young, our parents had lived a delicate balancing act in which Mom did all the cooking and Dad did all the driving. What would happen, we worried, if one of them were to become truly incapacitated?

It wasn't long before Dad turned the car keys over to us. Tuesday became the day, each week, when either my sisters or I would pick our parents up and accompany them to our mother's regular doctor appointment, which was near my home. When it was my turn, I would sometimes bring my parents back to my house after the morning appointment. After eating lunch—tuna melts—

we would all play with my toddler, Daniel, while Juliana was at school. While I enjoyed this "special time," as we called it, with my parents and Daniel, I also grumbled to myself about having to chauffeur Mom and Dad around with growing frequency. Having left my job to take care of my children, I was striving to develop a home-based consulting practice. With the demands of my kids, and now my parents, I could hardly find the time to get it off the ground.

Things only became worse. Concern for our parents turned into dismay as our mother developed a fatal blood disorder and our father's disorientation worsened to the level of Alzheimer's. Mom took a serious fall from which she never really recovered, and Dad eventually needed round-the-clock supervision for dementia.

For more than six years, my sisters and I went full throttle managing our parents' care, chaperoning each of them through harrowing trials filled with hospitals and doctors, injuries and infections, nursing homes, walkers, and wheelchairs. Making small talk in the car, eating tuna melts, and playing with Daniel's toy trucks together eventually seemed like the good old days.

During those years, of course, the age gap that had always differentiated my life from my sisters' was still apparent, perhaps more so than ever before. As Lois was planning her children's weddings and Cindy was putting her kids through college, my days were mostly spent nurturing my young children and struggling to grow my business. But when it came to assisting our ailing parents, Lois, Cindy, and I shouldered the responsibilities fairly equally. We each called doctors, ran errands, and refilled the pill boxes. We also took turns meeting Mom or Dad at the hospital at three or four o'clock in the morning, bleary eyed and shaking from the middle-of-the-night phone calls that had become routine.

Later, the three of us sat together at each parent's bedside as the end grew near. Our mother passed away in 2011, and our father in 2013.

***

Throughout the difficult years my sisters and I spent caring for our parents, I suspected something was out of balance. For the first time in our lives, Lois and Cindy had no wisdom to offer me, and I had none to follow. Unlike getting married and having children, riding the roller coaster of our parents' slow decline was the first life-occurrence all three of us were forced to muddle through *in real time*. We each struggled mightily, relying on the support of our families, our friends, and each other to cope with the many ups and downs. But rather than my more experienced siblings guiding me along, this was the blind leading the blind.

And on the spring morning when our father died in

his nursing home bed, so frail and weak he was nearly unrecognizable, my relationship with my sisters was transformed forever. As we sat holding Dad's hands and softly saying goodbye to him, Lois, Cindy and I were joined in an unfamiliar way. No longer trailing behind my sisters, I entered the next stage of life—that of parentless adulthood—at precisely the same moment they did. Not by age, but by the ordeal we had endured, and by our simultaneous loss and grief . . . I had caught up to them.

***

The years since my parents passed have been a mix of sadness and joy. While I'm blessed with a wonderful and healthy father-in-law, life without my own parents has become an odd reality. I sometimes experience a lonely pause late in the afternoon, when I used to reach for the phone to chat with Mom. Seeing my friends laughing with their parents on the beach, or multi-generational families eating together at the local diner, can spur quiet envy. I just can't help but notice, with the tiniest bit of resentment, that most people my age still have a parent or two to joke around with. Mostly, I miss my parents' doting love for me, and for my growing children.

Yet while my sisters and I miss Mom and Dad, the circle of life has continued for our family. Lois' two children each had babies of their own and named them lovingly in memory of our parents. My children have matured as well. Juliana celebrated her Sweet 16, and Daniel will soon start middle school. With the burden of caring for my parents now lifted, my consulting practice and career are thriving as well.

"Mom—you'll never believe this!" Juliana squealed recently, bounding through the front door and collapsing into a chair after her first hour-long driving lesson. "The driving instructor was asking about my family—he knows Auntie Loey!"

"No kidding?" I asked, bewildered. "How so?"

Juliana explained that the instructor, his wife, and Lois were all childhood friends.

"He and his wife remember you, too," Juliana continued. "He called his wife from the car and said, 'I'm driving with the baby's daughter.' She knew exactly who he meant."

The Baby. Clearly, I'm a legend.

I chuckle knowing I will be forever young to many people. But just as surely, my self-image has shifted ever so slightly since my parents' passing, and this change has been largely positive. I have realized that, although my sisters can't always walk me through difficult situations, their companionship on this unpaved road of life gives me strength to weather the journey. And truth be told, the subtle parity I now feel with them has given me a new, grown-up confidence I never really had before.

"My sister, my friend…" read the caption on a birthday card with pretty pink roses, our mother's favorite.

Ah, that's the one, I concluded. Friends, yes. Always.

Amy Halzel Willis' creative writing has appeared in publications ranging from the Boston Herald, *to the* Brandeis Magazine, *to* Covenant of the Generations: New Prayers, Poems and Meditations from Women of Reform Judaism. *Amy is also a consultant writer specializing in grant proposals, reports, articles, and websites. With a background in health care and public policy, Amy helps clients from across the health care, non-profit, and business communities to achieve their goals through clear, organized writing. Amy's website, www.amywilliswriting. com, describes her business and contains links to her published pieces. Amy lives in Needham, Massachusetts, with her husband and two children.*

TIME TURNS BACK ON ITSELF
By Laura Grace Weldon

"He fit right into the palm of my hand," my mother says again. Her arm trembles now when she holds it out. "His head here," she gestures to her fingertips, "his little bottom here, and his legs curled up at my wrist. They never gave poor patients the incubators. They said babies that small didn't make it anyway. But he looked right at me, and I knew he would live. I held him every night in the nursery until he was discharged. I wish I knew what happened to him."

My mother's stories of her early years as a registered nurse are becoming more frequent. I settle back and listen, encouraging her with my questions. The house seems darker each time I visit, curtains drawn against the daylight, although the family photos on every surface still fade in their frames. The cluttered rooms are hard to recognize as the same ones from my childhood. Time seems to stretch and bend out of proportion on these long afternoons.

"I nearly died of a staph infection when I was in nurses' training," says my mother as she starts another story. "It was all through my bloodstream. The doctors were amazed I pulled through." She shakes her head. "It was a miracle."

My two teenaged sons come in from doing yard work. They wash their hands, eat the snack she loves to offer them, and politely chat with her. She has tales to tell them, too, usually emphasizing the value of working hard and saving money. Today she asks them to retrieve a bit of laundry she can't reach. Somehow, it sailed over the washing machine lid to fall somewhere behind the washer. Tossing anything while hanging on to a walker is an accomplishment for someone whose movements are as uncertain as hers.

I thought I'd heard all her stories, yet she tells the boys her laundry throw probably stems from her teen years when she used to be quite the softball pitcher.

"I never was much of a runner in gym, but I had a great throwing arm."

"You never told me that, Mom!" I say.

"There's plenty I haven't told you," she says. Her gaze drifts, as though her mind is time-traveling back sixty years ago to that field of high school girls.

My father doesn't settle down for long conversations during these visits. He likes to work in the yard with his grandchildren, making use of their youthful energy, while my mother and I talk. I go outside to spend ten or fifteen minutes with him, reveling in the quieter connection we share, fully aware my mother waits for me to return through the full length of each minute I'm away from her.

I see my parents bridging the passage beyond old age in their own ways. Always thinking ahead, my father redesigns the garden and invents odd labor-saving devices. My mother looks back, revisiting her stronger years. I'm greedy for time. I want decades more with my parents despite their poor health. Their tradition of waving goodbye at the door as I back the car out always brings tears to my eyes.

***

On the long drive home, my 16-year-old son comes across an old Emerson, Lake, and Palmer tune, "From the Beginning," on the radio. Time twists around itself again. I recall listening to this record in the late seventies from the same house we just left, although the raspberry-hued carpet of my girlhood bedroom is now hidden under a pile of boxes. I used to climb out the window of that bedroom and lay on the pebbly roof, looking at the stars. I paid such close attention to the music of my teens that I felt wrapped inside the notes and lyrics: *You see it's all clear. You were meant to be here.*

While the song plays, I remember being a wispy 14-year-old who bought batik scarves from the forbidden head shop in town. I twisted them into halter tops, which I wore under more demure shirts until I was safely out of the house. I'd tell my parents I was going to see a girlfriend when I was really meeting my boyfriend. He and I kissed so much I was surprised my mother didn't notice my swollen and reddened lips on my return. When the song ends, I'm almost startled to find myself driving a car—a woman in her forties accompanied by two nearly grown children.

As time turns back on itself in our memories, it reshapes us. It occurs to me I loved Emerson, Lake, and Palmer because they honored two sounds I couldn't imagine converging. I'd rejected my parents' religion and with it the evocative strains of organ music. Instead, I spent my babysitting money on albums with what I considered more soul-stirring sounds. Emerson, Lake, and Palmer put hymns and rock together for me.

As I head south with my boys, I feel my face lifted to the sky again. I try to say something to my kids about how odd time and memory can be. But they're young and the radio dial needs flipping. I guess we're bridging our own passages. I take a breath, choosing to hold on to the peace of this moment so this exact car ride with my sons will always feel as close to me as the palm of my own hand.

Laura Grace Weldon lives on Bit of Earth Farm where she's an editor and marginally useful farm wench. She's the author of a poetry collection Tending *and a handbook of alternative education,* Free Range Learning. *Her work appears in the* Christian Science Monitor, *Wired.com, Geez, Lilipoh, Mom Egg Review, J Journal, the Shine Journal, Musie Pie Press, L'Initiation, Pudding House, and others. Connect with her at lauragraceweldon.com*

THE WEIGHT OF FRIDAYS
By Kelly Garriott Waite

"You know," Dad said from his hospital bed just after his lung biopsy, "if you get philosophical about it, the bucket list is fairly complete." He looked into my eyes and the eyes of my sister and gave a brief nod before his own eyes filled with tears.

We would wait several days for a diagnosis. But we all knew that he had cancer; that the masses in his brain picked up in an MRI the Monday before had metastasized from the ominous spots on his lungs.

Dad agreed to a course of radiation: fifteen days of treatment that would leave his mouth and throat sore, his head aching, his brain swollen. My siblings and I set up a schedule: Mondays, the oldest sister would head to the farm, drive with Mom and Dad to treatment, and spend the night. Wednesdays, the middle sister would do the same. Fridays fell to me. Our brother would drive into town as he could, spending several days at a time at the farm. We exchanged dozens of text messages every day:

"Can someone print out a HIPAA form and bring it out?"

"Dad's being discharged from the hospital Friday."

"I'm bringing dinner."

That first weekend, steeled by loud rock music and a cup of Venti Starbucks coffee bought on the turnpike, I drove home, blinking back tears as I turned in the driveway. I went into the den, walked to the La-Z-Boy, where Dad would spend the majority of the rest of his life, and planted a kiss on his cheek, something I hadn't done in years.

In several hours of recorded interviews I conducted with him, Dad told me about his childhood. He told me about milking the cows at his grandparents' farm and delivering post office packages on his pony named Duke. He told me about coming home from the Army and visiting his elderly grandmother. He spoke of the long silences between them; how he listened to the ticking clock, feeling that the visit would never come to an end.

On the sixth day of radiation, Dad called his treatment off. He wanted to die. He wanted to die at home. The tenor of the texts my siblings and I exchanged changed:

"Hospice is coming Friday."

"What will Medicare cover?"

"I'm bringing a walker."

Quietly, my mother, siblings, and I speculated as to how much time Dad had remaining. A year? Six months? We had no idea, although the doctor had told us that the five radiation treatments had bought him—and us—some time.

But Dad didn't want time. He wanted to die immediately. He asked a hospice nurse to, for lack of a better word, "speed things up," to "euthanize" him, as the nurse bluntly put it, denying his request.

Why the rush to die? It could've been those brain tumors, crowding out what my family considered rational thought. It could've been that Dad considered himself a burden to his family. Maybe he didn't want his wife and children to see him going messily through his final journey. Or perhaps Dad, who never went to sleep without tomorrow's to-do list sketched out, wanted to die on his own terms.

But I fear that my father, as an aging, terminally ill man, felt useless. Unimportant. Unseen.

***

What did we do, Dad and I, the following Friday as the cancer was given free rein to chew through his brain? As the cells in his lungs crowded out his ability to breathe? How did he and I pass the time when we knew his time on earth was near its end? We went through a box of mementoes he'd stashed in a cabinet: his children's report cards, hand-made Father's Day cards, pictures of the family business. We rummaged through decades-old photographs. We continued our interviews. At one point, when the recorder was off, Dad tearfully told me he had no regrets.

After three weeks, our interviews came to an end. Watching Dad sitting in his easy chair, folding into himself, staring at the TV or sleeping, his mouth gaping open, waiting for the end, felt sad. Wrong. Too much for a person—for him? for his family?—to bear. I suddenly became a believer in a person's right to die, something to which I'd never before given much thought. I had dreams in which I set a bottle of pills beside my father's table, giving him a knowing look as I left the room.

Dad progressively grew weaker. More withdrawn. The texts between my siblings and me changed again:

"Dad fell today."

"He doesn't look good."

"We're upping his meds."

I soon began to dread Fridays. I was tired of giving up my weekends. Tired of being tired. Tired, most of all, of coming face-to-face with the truth of Dad's death. Every Friday I'd see how much closer to dying he was. Too, I dreaded Fridays, because without the recorder running between us, without the list of questions in my lap, I no longer knew what to say. The silences became deeper. More regular.

One Friday, Dad consumed a dozen cookies, each slathered in butter. He ate ice cream. Donuts. Sweet rolls. The next Friday—the Friday I failed to kiss him, the last Friday I saw him alive—I sat on the couch as Dad slept, listening to the ticking of the clock and the silence of the room. By now, Dad was barely eating, barely smoking, barely communicating. He hardly ever had the TV on.

Yet he continued to fall. Despite the fact that he was now, at his request, wearing diapers, Dad insisted on regularly going to the bathroom, often just to smoke, making his way across the den's rug, his metal walker creaking with every step as he headed across the dining room, through the kitchen and into the mudroom's half bathroom.

The days were long. How should I fill them now that I couldn't hide behind my notepad? I helped prepare meals. I got Dad endless glasses of ice water to soothe his throat. I administered medication. I stared, with my mother, at the birds gathering outside the kitchen window visiting the many feeders Mom and Dad had placed there over the years. I reminded Dad again and again what day it was, and what time. I explained, as he stared out into the afternoon sunshine, that it wasn't yet time for bed.

Evenings, I watched movies on Netflix with my mom as Dad nodded off. We woke him at eleven o'clock to give him the medicines that, by all rights, should've kept him comfortable and calm during the night. But while we slept, Dad grew agitated, overcoming morphine, a sleeping pill, two tablets of Percogesic, and an anti-anxiety pill to rise several times throughout the night to go to the bathroom.

That Friday—the Friday I failed to kiss him on the cheek—Dad fell again, shortly after we'd gone to bed. The fire department arrived, lights flashing. Hospice came to check Dad's vitals. I listened to the suggestions to keep Dad from falling: Tie a bell to his walker. Get up every hour to take him to the bathroom. Put a baby monitor next to his chair. I knew then that Mom could no longer be alone with my father, that he needed continual assistance to and from the bathroom, that we'd have to rise whenever he did, so that he wouldn't fall again.

I texted my sister: "I'll stay another night. Can you take the next two?"

We learned to haul Dad from his chair, one arm each hooked beneath his armpits while he struggled to stand with the help of his walker. We stood on either side of him as he made his way across the den rug into the dining room, through the kitchen and finally—*finally*—into the bathroom where we'd wrestle him onto the toilet. When he was done, we'd assist him back into his chair, promising him again and again, as he struggled to sit, that we wouldn't let him fall. We tucked the blankets around him and went back to bed, knowing at any moment, he might try to rise again.

That last weekend, something shifted in me. As I took Dad his meager meals on a wooden tray, then fed him from a spoon or held a drinking glass to his mouth; as I saw his skinny white legs, his bottom covered in a diaper; as I wiped the drool from his face; as I popped blue pills into his compliant birdy mouth and gazed into his trusting, tired blue eyes, my heart broke open: I learned to see Dad more deeply. I learned to be more patient. More kind. Compassionate.

Dad's death was certainly not pretty; every day, his beard grew thicker. White sores developed along his gumline and lips. His dentures jutted from his mouth. His hair stood up. His pants slipped down. His toenails grew into claws. Yes, Dad's death was not pretty. And yet, it was a beautiful thing.

***

Just six weeks after being diagnosed, my father died. Every day, I stand at my kitchen window, staring at the birds visiting my new feeders. My days are filled with silence. No text updates jangle at my nerves. No telephone calls send chills up my spine. Once again, my weekends belong to me.

How I wish that were not so.

Kelly Garriott Waite writes essays and fiction from Ohio. Her work has appeared in the Globe and Mail, *the* Philadelphia Inquirer, *the* Christian Science Monitor, *the* Woven Tale Press Selected Works 2015, *and elsewhere. She's currently researching the lives of both her great-grandfather, a Polish immigrant, and the second owner of her historic home, an English immigrant adopted into the Chickasaw Nation.*

SHAPES IN THE CLOUDS
By Pamela Valentine

My grandfather moved in with us the summer I turned 11. My father sat down at dinner one night and announced he was bringing two more people into a three-bedroom house that already held five. My sister threw a fit and refused, outright, to give up her room, before stomping off down the hall and slamming the door. My brother shrugged and went back to eating. The news changed nothing for him.

When my father's eyes fell on me, his youngest, I smiled and said I couldn't wait until he got here and offered to move into the basement so he could use my room. My easy acceptance surprised my dad, but I shared a bedroom wall with my parents and knew the real reason behind the move.

My grandfather was sick. Senile dementia, I heard my dad say. Possibly Alzheimer's. This was the eighties and they could only confirm the latter postmortem. In the light of the narrow beam of my flashlight, I paged through the dictionary and encyclopedias, learning what I could about those words. His wife needed help caring for him, living independently was no longer an option. But none of the nursing homes they applied to would take him, now that he'd been diagnosed.

My parents fought about the decision. My mother cried. We couldn't possibly fit my grandfather and his wife in here. Why couldn't his sisters take them? All their children were grown, they had bigger houses, extra bathrooms.

My dad remained firm. He was the only son, the youngest child, and it was his duty and his pleasure to bring his father into his home. We would manage, somehow.

He moved in days after the announcement. He was practically a stranger to me. His wife, Grace, was a battleship: a former nurse, a former school principal, a former nun. They'd married a few short years after my grandmother passed away, for companionship. She took over cleaning, cooking, and praying for our whole family, and tended to her tasks diligently, if somewhat righteously.

Grandpa was the quiet poet, the introvert, the thinker. He walked every day, smoking the cigarettes that were banned inside the house. I walked with him whenever I could, partly because I was tasked by my parents to make sure he didn't get lost, but mostly because I loved to listen to him talk.

He told stories about the railyards where he worked, about my dad as a little boy, about my grandmother, who died when I was 3 and who everyone said I was so much like. He pointed out brilliantly feathered birds and shapes in the clouds and fluffy-tailed squirrels as they hopped from tree to tree. He asked me what I saw and what I thought and about things that mattered to me.

His conversations rambled and wound their way from one subject to the next. Sometimes he knew me, knew my name, and knew why I was there. Sometimes he'd grow very confused and frightened; he'd stumble to a stop in the middle of the sidewalk, and turn in a circle, trying to find his way.

I was always there to take his arm and lead him home and tell him it'd be okay.

And for a little while, it was okay.

The second winter brought pneumonia, and with it the discovery of a tumor on his lung. I no longer shared a bedroom wall with my parents, but I knew it was terminal. I knew from the way my father told us Grandpa was coming home from the hospital that December, and I knew there would be nurses and machines and he wouldn't be able to get out of bed. My dad didn't talk about the treatments or chemotherapy that I read about in books at the library. He talked about hospice, about making Grandpa comfortable, about quality of life. And he did it in a hushed voice, near tears.

I sat by Grandpa's side every day after school that winter. He taught me how to speak Polish and how to do crossword puzzles and how to play pinochle. I wrote him poems and sang him songs and drew pictures that made him laugh.

Other days he grew agitated and angry and confused. He'd thrash around on his bed and pull out his catheter and IV and scream to be let out. The hospice nurse and Grace would race into the room and push me aside. Sometimes he'd scream at me from the doorway to help him, to get him out. Other times he'd scream at me to leave him alone.

My father tried to talk to me about what was going on with Grandpa. We had to understand he was sick. We had to forgive him for the way he was acting. We had to try to remember he still loved us and cared about us and to not be frightened. Only, I wasn't frightened, never. I'd read enough about Alzheimer's disease by then to know it was the disease, and not my grandfather, saying those things.

He died that spring, in April. He passed away quietly, alone, moments after I left the room to head to church to sing in the choir on Good Friday. I wasn't even 13 years old.

***

I missed him. I still miss him. I spent my teenage years comparing him to my dad, trying to find any likeness, any similarity, any sign of the gentle man I grew to love in my childhood. I railed against the unfairness that left me with a father I viewed as ignorant and uneducated and loud. I grew resentful of the fact that my grandfather, my humble, creative, quiet grandfather had raised *him* and not *me*. I felt like the universe had played a great cosmic joke on us all.

My dad and I spent my early twenties fighting, screaming, crying, raging at each other and my late twenties avoiding each other, almost altogether. Somehow, I transformed all the grief I felt over my grandfather's death into a knife of accusation against my father. Attacking him for not doing more. For not finding better treatments or taking him to better doctors. For not keeping him alive longer.

I forgot about the fights my parents had, over money usually, because there was never enough. I forgot about the canned veggies we ate every dinner and the powdered milk we adjusted to drinking, because we couldn't afford more. I forgot about Hungry Jack mashed potatoes and lemon pepper seasoning and all the other culinary tricks my parents used to make us forget we were eating on a budget.

I forgot about desperately hopping around outside the bathroom, because we only had one to share, and I forgot the late nights and weekends my dad spent putting in a new toilet, by himself, into a closet of our house. I forgot about sleeping on a mattress on the floor of an unfinished basement during a thunderstorm and waking up soaking wet and shivering because the sump pump gave out. And

I forgot how my father finished the basement that fall, so we had four walls and a door and our own bedroom.

I forgot about the doctor visits, the hospital stays, the blood tests and x-rays and MRIs and CT scans. I forgot the work my parents had to miss, the vacation and sick time they had to use, to take Grandpa to his appointments. And I forgot about the way my father wept when he took me in his arms to tell me his father had died.

And I blamed him for bringing Grandpa into my life in the first place, thinking, foolishly, had I never known that gentle soul, I would've been spared so much loss. My father gave me the gift of his father, and I tried to wrap it up in blame and regret.

***

I gave birth to my oldest when I was 30 and named him after my grandfather. It made my father cry. When we visit now, most of the time is spent listening to my dad talk. Rambling and winding and twisting through memories, sometimes repeating himself and sometimes petering off without any real point.

My father is now the same age my grandpa was the year he moved in. They look so much alike. The same deep blue eyes, soft papery skin with liver spots, and *the hands*. I notice the resemblance most in the hands; my father's hands are gentle now, like Grandpa's were.

My father smells of ivory soap and outdoors, instead

of Grandpa's cigarettes and the deeper, bittersweet smell of sickness. But he talks about jobs he did and places he worked, about his childhood a lot, but mostly, about his wife and kids. He points out roof shingles and siding and gutters, instead of birds and squirrels and shapes in the clouds, but I feel the presence of my grandfather in those simple things. I hear the echo of his gentle voice and his soft chuckle and the love that has been there all along.

In those moments, I see the little boy my grandfather loved so dearly, the young man that made him so proud, the father that tried so hard to live up to his own father. In those moments, I feel the weight of my father's decision to watch his father die, to live through that grief and tragedy while helping his own children do the same.

In those moments, I wonder if I'll have the strength to do the same, if the time comes. And it's my father's voice that answers inside my heart, that says I'm his youngest, and it would be my duty and my pleasure to bring my father into my home.

It's my father's strength that assures me, no matter how difficult it might seem, we'd manage somehow, and it's my grandfather's memory that holds me tight and lets me know it'll be okay.

Pamela Valentine shares the joys and challenges of raising a gender diverse child as Affirmed Mom through ChicagoNow. She was recently awarded a BlogHer 2016 Voices of the Year Award and second place for Excellence in Blogging from the National Gay and Lesbian Journalists Association. Her essays have been featured on Scary Mommy; Cosmo; Good Housekeeping; *Brain, Child Magazine; and in the Her Stories anthology,* So Glad They Told Me.

AIR SUPPLY
By Kristie Betts Letter

I have a speech of fire, that fain would blaze,
But that this folly drowns it.
(Hamlet IV.vii.190-191)

It was an Air Supply song—that much we agree on. But which one? I remember singing "Making Love Out of Nothing At All" and my husband swears it was "All Out of Love." Either way, we all belted the lyrics like Christmas Eve carols, filling the car with music on road trips. Almost shouting.

With Mom in the final stages of cancer and a new baby, we didn't take many road trips that fall. One Saturday, the baby was on the floor in the living room crawling all over my husband, Bobby, when the Air Supply song came on and Bobby started to sing. The baby clearly loved the slow dance music of the eighties and began to kick rhythmically, smiling. An Air Supply fan! I plopped down beside them on the beige carpet and began to sing along.

Then Mom came down to the floor, too. She did a sort of a roll out of her wheelchair and landed next to us. Though she often couldn't remember common words or our names, somewhere in her head, tucked behind the brain tumors, the lyrics of this particular song remained.

We sang Air Supply. All of us. Even the baby tried to sing along, yelping as we all sprawled on the floor.

Sure, it took both my husband and me to get Mom back into her wheelchair, but this moment shone as a happy one in the dark days before my mother died.

***

My mother held on long past the point when anyone thought she would or possibly could. Her spine curved, her face expanded, and her hands shook incessantly. They injected her with chemotherapy's poison to prolong her life, but she couldn't move through the world or remember what her favorite foods were called. By the time she sang that Air Supply song with us on the floor, she sometimes ate things that weren't food at all. I had to hide the bath beads. She mistook their brightly colored globes for candy every time.

When friends and family arrived to see her after the cancer treatments began, they had to control their reactions. Mom didn't look anything like herself, or anything resembling "normal" for that matter. Her body bent, her cheeks swelled, and her head was bald as an egg. Children stared while slowly backing away. It was that bad.

"Why does she sound like that?" they'd ask. "Should we call the doctor?" Our visitors, the ones who hadn't been here for the progression of symptoms, panicked at the sound of the Darth Vader rasp of Mom's breathing. They gasped at her baldness and swollen cheeks. They jumped out of their chairs when they saw her shuffle/lurch in an attempt to move with her cancer-mangled bones. When asked about her condition, I didn't go into detail about what the hospice nurses told us various symptoms meant (lungs filling with fluid, body shutting down, brain being destroyed), only that this was the "new normal" as we approached the undiscovered country.

She started calling me "Mom." As her body fell apart, time did too. Those neat chronologies that separate the living from the dead, the possible from the impossible blurred and fell away. My husband and I simultaneously cared for a baby learning to communicate with the world around her and for my mother whose lines of communication were closing. Time folded in on itself. Nearing the end of days, we hoped there were enough wrinkles or rips in time for Mom. A door to Narnia might've allowed us to slip away and spend years together while only a few seconds passed in the work-day world. Only songs from stronger days opened the door to the past, a moment beyond the body and its invaders.

The hospice nurse explained "transition"— a process by which the body systematically shuts down as the person prepares for death. The nurse was calm, patient, saintly. Like a preschool teacher. She was used to dealing with people who weren't putting logic first.

The nurse went to her car and returned with the last straw, the kicker—adult-sized diapers. Huge. Massive. *Pink*. I'm sure the color was for easy reference as to whether or not the particular tablecloth-sized diaper was for a man or a woman, but the pastel color suggested nothing more than a preposterously large baby. My husband and I stared down in horror as the nurse modeled how to put a diaper on a fully-grown woman.

Parenting was one thing. This was something else entirely.

"So, you just roll her to the side and slide it under," the nurse continued.

We both had a hard time paying attention to the diaper demonstration. Mom now sat within earshot.

That, above anything else, told me this was the end.

If Mom had been able to process what was going on, she would've been horrified, would've stood up from her wheelchair and raged with a speech of fire. She would've cursed and burned down the house before she allowed those mega-Pampers anywhere near her. "I hope I die before anyone changes my diapers," my mother had said to me when we first found out she was ill. When hospice nurses asked her about the end of life wishes, she'd repeated that sentiment. But now, in the last gasps, she had no more words to offer. We could've raged for her, I guess. We could've refused the diapers. My husband and I could've gently pressed the pillow on her face then and there, ending the supply of air as she had asked us to do, before any of us realized what that would mean.

"Do we have a responsibility to kill her?" I asked my husband.

He took several seconds before saying, "I hope not." We had let her down. But neither of us was up for a mercy killing of the woman we loved so much. We played songs that rewound in time, to my mother drunk-dancing at our wedding, singing while she cooked dinner, shaking with excitement (still) about the Beatles.

When Mom lost the meaning of specific words, the music remained. She remembered the lyrics, and we could still sing together. Her air supply dwindled. As our baby learned to say words, my mother forgot them, moving in the opposite direction. So while teaching a baby to grasp a spoon and listen to words, the midwifing of death entered the same space, and only the music bound us all together.

"Mom refused to put on pajamas or the diapers. I tried to tell her she's been wearing the same thing for two days, but I gave up. I put the diaper beneath her on the bed," I said to my husband.

"Don't worry too much about that stuff," Bobby said. "There's only so much you can do." He put his arm around me.

"You are the only thing keeping me sane," I said, snuggling closer.

"Then I'm an abject failure, sweetie," he said, with a kiss that took my breath away.

My husband put on music, the only thing that can ease having a parent die at home. Loud, loud music.

Kristie Betts Letter's work has appeared in The Massachusetts Review, The North Dakota Quarterly, Washington Square, Passages North, Pangolin Papers, *and* The Southern Humanities Review. *Her novel* Snow and White *was just picked up by KT Literary. She's won several teaching awards for forcing Hamlet on high school seniors, and also plays a mean game of pub trivia, where she never misses a question about the eighties. Kristiebettsletter.com or @kristieletter.*

SOUNDS OF LOVE AND LIFE
By Kim Love Stump

I.

"Rolls, cornbread, or hushpuppies?" Faye asks in a rush, pen poised above the order pad.

"Uh . . . what did I just order?" my dad queries Faye.

He's not kidding, and Faye doesn't miss a beat. "Baked ham," she replies.

"Oh, whole wheat toast then, dry."

It's been months since I've heard him order anything but whole wheat toast, which always arrives dry whether he remembers to order it that way or not. I'm here only once a week for a single meal, but ever since my mother died, he eats here roughly ten times that often. He used to order cornbread occasionally and hushpuppies, those small, deep-fried cornmeal cakes, frequently. But now he seems to be in a loop of dry toast. Perhaps it's the regularity of that small change that's impacted his blood sugar numbers. They're consistently lower recently, even though he'll eat dessert after lunch—as always—and again after dinner—as always.

Before Faye hustles over to take our order, moving faster than you might expect for her age, Cindy arrives with our black coffee and ice water with lemon, not much ice. His constancy has the waitresses trained. The routine continues. When lunch arrives, the ham has already been cut for him in large bite-size pieces, and there's twice as much as anyone else in the laminate-boothed diner is served.

"That Doug, he sure looks after me." Daddy says as he grins and starts in on his coleslaw. "Best $200 I ever spent," he continues, "Did I ever tell you that story?"

Before he can tell me, *again,* about the guy threatening Doug (the cook) in the parking lot and Daddy stopping to ask what was wrong and Doug explaining his inability to pay his $200 debt and Daddy pulling out his expensive alligator wallet (the latest edition of the ones mother gave him for Christmas every couple of years when his became worn at the corners) and Daddy giving two hundred-dollar bills to the guy threatening Doug and then saying, "Now leave this boy the hell alone!"—I quickly say, "Yes, that was a good deed that really paid off."

I check my cell phone, *again,* hoping for a witty text from my son, a sophomore at the University of North Carolina at Chapel Hill, or an exuberant email from my daughter finishing her last year at University of Virginia, but there's nothing alerting me to a welcome distraction.

I eat my salad—iceberg, cheap grated cheddar, decently grilled chicken breast, and the best tomatoes I'll have all summer—and begin a story about Stuart, my daughter with my dad's name, but I can see Daddy's gaze slide off my face to a more distant locale over my shoulder. Behind his glasses, tears slowly well in both his eyes, though only one has sight—the other is a very good prosthetic—as he watches a husband navigate his wife's wheelchair to the table next to ours. I stop the story. He doesn't notice.

I recapture his attention, and we navigate the remainder of lunch with a discussion of the weather and which errands we'll do after lunch.

"I'm going to run to the restroom while you pay," I say after he finishes the last of his "chocolate delite." I don't need eyes in the back of my head to see Daddy struggle to his feet, put two single bills from the money clip in his front pocket on the table, and walk with his oddly stiff gate to the counter where he'll sit down on a bar stool and pay for our lunch. The pattern is entrenched.

I return as Faye is handing him his change, all the bills turned the same way, just like he does for himself if another of the waitresses—Angela, Panzi, Cindy or Sherry—give him his bills turned every which way. I ask Faye about her health; she was out last week with heart palpitations, but all is well now, and I say goodbye and turn to leave, thinking we've safely concluded another lunch.

But as I push the door open and turn to remind Daddy to watch the threshold, I see he's looking again at the wife in the wheelchair. His eyes dampen and fill again, his chin trembles, "If that had been your mother . . ." he starts, but has to stop. "She would've rather it happened the way it did than to be like that," he says sadly as he steps out into the September heat.

The truth or falsehood of his statement eludes me. I don't reply.

II.

I'm hardly out of the driveway when my phone rings. It's my father. I recognize the ringtone.

"Hey, honey," my dad says.

"Hey, Daddy, I'm sorry I missed your call earlier."

"What did I call for?"

"I don't know, you didn't leave a message," I say in response.

"Oh . . . right. I couldn't. Your phone said your mailbox was full."

"Really? It shouldn't be. But thanks; I'll check it right now. Love you, see you Thursday."

"Ok. Bye. Love you. See you Thursday."

Sigh. I hang up, frustrated; I still don't know why my father called earlier in the day, and I'm confused over why my new phone's voicemail would be full already. I didn't realize all the messages from my old phone would transfer over. In anticipation of losing them and in a fit of extreme sentimentality, I had transferred a bunch of saved voice messages that I couldn't part with to a CD, a permanent record of my family's and friends' voices.

As I drive out of the neighborhood, I speed dial my voice inbox and delete the two new hang-up calls someone, presumably my dad, left there. The automated voice then says I have thirty-eight saved messages. The thirty-eight I had so carefully saved.

"Hey momma—it's me," my daughter's then-high-school-senior voice chirps in my ear. "I just wanted to call and say 'thank you.' Thank you for all you do. I couldn't possibly do it without you. You're the best! I love you!" I smile and press 9 to save the message, *again*, rationalizing I can keep a few messages from my family on this new phone to have near me.

I have a good idea of what will follow: a voice message from my dear friend Ruth, a smile in her voice telling me she's booked a dinner reservation for my husband and me in her new hometown of Raleigh. I decide to delete that one, confident the CD holding all thirty-eight messages is safely stored back at the house in my office.

Next, it's Betsy, my best friend here in Charlotte, asking me where I am. The Y or Laughing Buddha is her guess. It was a good guess at the time she left the message, but I haven't been to Laughing Buddha in probably three years. That's how old some of these messages are. I delete that one, too.

The message after that is from my son. "Hey Mom," his then-junior-in-high-school voice rumbles. "I saw you called, wanted to say 'Hi,' and let you know I won't be here later tonight—I'm going to a party. Oh, and your friend, Sherry? Sherry Hasting, or something like that, called and asked me to go to church? Anyway, I don't know who that is. Talk to you later. I love you." Even three years later, I feel thankful for *Sheree's* offer to take my reticent son to church when she was visiting Chattanooga and he was in boarding school. I can't bring myself to delete the message.

Next, a message from Mom. "Hey, babe. I'm on my way to get my hair done. If I'm not home when you get there, I'll be back around noon. I love you." I carefully listen to the instructions to press 7 to erase and 9 to save to make absolutely sure I don't erase my dead mother's voice from my phone. *Can she possibly be dead when I've just heard her sweet voice talk to me?* I ask myself as I press the 9 key on my phone.

Following that is my husband telling me he's landed somewhere or another, maybe it was New York or Los Angeles or Hong Kong, that he loves me, that he'll call me later. I erase it without much thought, knowing there are another dozen similar messages among the thirty-eight. The next three messages are more from my mom.

I'll keep a copy of these on this phone, too.

"Hey babe. I'm back home from the beauty shop. See you when you get here. Drive carefully. I love you." She sounds so well. I know she was already sick when she left the message, her cough already chronic, her colon cancer already stage IV, having metastasized to her liver and omentum.

"Hey babe," she has a smile in her voice. "I just wondered which plan you decided to follow. I'll see you when you get here." I've already forgotten what plans she might've been talking about. Probably whether I was coming prepared to spend the night or whether I was making the hour-and-a-half trip from Charlotte to Asheboro as just a day trip. "Call me when you get this." I wish I could. I dialed her number once accidentally after she died. It already had been reassigned to a man with a nice voice but no acquaintance with my mother. "I love you," she concludes.

"Hey babe, I woke up and you weren't in the room. I just wondered where you were," she sounds tired and sick. She was. I can't take anymore. I end the call to my voicemail inbox.

For whatever reason, I put up my left hand to cup my face. I'm crying. As I sit in my car waiting for the left turn signal to change, I reach across the empty passenger seat for the Bible that I keep in my car. The cover is warm to my touch as I flip the pages to Philippians 4:8— . . ."whatever is true, whatever is honorable, whatever is right, whatever is pure, whatever is lovely, whatever is of good repute, if there is any excellence and if anything worthy of praise, let your mind dwell on these things."

It's a talisman verse, a reorientation for my thoughts. I wrote a devotional for church on it once, somehow tying in the idea of butterflies. I look up in the direction of the stoplight, but something else catches my eye. A single butterfly, bright yellow and small, flutters across the busy intersection. Something lovely, something worthy of praise.

I wipe the tears off my face, put the Bible in the seat beside me, and drive on as the light turns green.

III.

I know we were in South Myrtle Beach, and I know it was summer. I remember I was cocooned in my grandmother's arms on the screened porch of a small beach house one row back from the ocean. As we rocked, she softly sang "Hush Little Baby" to me in the dark, while adult conversation washed around us. For the others sitting with us, the song was probably just another background noise—like the crickets, like the hoot owl, like the distant splash of waves. But for me, the lullaby assured all will be right with the world, even when the world doesn't work the way you expect, because someone who loves you is going to make sure of it.

My grandfather rocked beside us, and my mother and father swayed in a softly creaking porch swing. The air felt cool and my soft nylon nightgown was as silky smooth as the tendril of hair I wrapped and rewrapped around my finger. Granny, my great-grandmother, was surely there, as was my youngest aunt, who nestled into the family tree between my age and my mother's. While my aunt was a sometimes playmate, I most often felt like she was running away from me, not content to play in the children's world of make believe my cousins and I invented, wanting, instead, to make her own fairytale world turn into a true story.

Why does this trip hold so vividly in my memories? I'm not sure. I was with these family members all the time in the day-to-day. Perhaps what made the memory adhere was that, instead of the constant call of work, with time for me squeezed in, there was a constant call to play, not to mention the store bought luxuries—cherry pie from the A&P grocery store, for example, resting in its white box with the clear, crinkly see-through top, showing fleshy filling and crispy crust. It was meant for after lunch, but on this trip, I was given a piece to eat for breakfast.

Or perhaps it was my first encounter with death that

seared this particular vacation in my mind. On a mid-morning walk to the beach, the hard-packed sand of the yard already burning through my small, rubber flip-flops, I held my daddy's hand and danced alongside his thin legs as we prepared to cross the asphalt. There, in the center of the two-lane beach road, lay a pile of white feathers. A bird. A seagull.

"What's wrong with it, Daddy? Why isn't it moving?"

"It's dead, sweetheart."

I don't know if I asked any more questions about death that trip. I did, though, later when my first dog, a happy beagle named Penny, died in an accident. "But she'll be back, won't she?" I asked my father. The answer, of course, was no. I cried. And so did he. There are some things even the best papas can't fix.

And now, all but one of those people who loved me so well on that summer vacation and throughout my childhood are gone, lost to heart attacks or old age or cancer or pneumonia. Only my aunt and I remain.

And I wonder, is it all right for her? Her dreams of marriage and a family never materialized. She burst forth from her cocoon but never really left it, mired and stuck by her concepts of obligation and love.

And what of me? Am I all right? On this fifteenth day of April, exactly five years after my father's death, am I all right with where I find myself? Strangely, I am. I live the life that is not the one I expected. I have the joy of loving and of being loved by other people: my husband, my children, my friends. That is, I suppose, my solution to the disappointments and surprising losses that life most certainly brings.

It's not what I expected. Perhaps that is the real underlying meaning of the song my grandmother softly sang to me on the screened porch of that small beach house so long ago. Life never is what we expect. But it is good, every precious moment of it.

Kim Love Stump has loved to read and write ever since she can remember. While fiction is her first writing love, she has written everything from equity recommendations for a bank trust department to Bible studies. She's also a frequent writer of memoir. Whether a snippet of real life or an intricate fantasy land from her series Journeys from Ayrden, *Kim loves world building through words. The real-life world she has built in Charlotte, North Carolina, she happily shares with her husband of thirty plus years, her two grown children and one son-in-law whenever they visit, and whichever friends are around to receive a dose of love and joy.*

STARS I WILL FIND
By Julia Tagliere

Some have asked me why we did what we did, why we didn't just leave him there, didn't let him hit the rocky bottomed abyss we'd kept him from for so long. I have only one answer: love. Not the kind of love most people think of, but ugly, raw, often one-sided love.

In the comfort of the darkened church, my daughter takes her place at the grand piano. I think how proud my father would be to see her, and when she plays the first soft notes of her piece, "Stars I Shall Find," the tears that have been strangling me for the last few days begin to flow.

***

My earliest memories of my father hum with the constant sound of his music. A gifted musician, my father collected organs and pianos the way other men collect cars: a nice habit, if you have the money, which my father never did. On Sundays, he woke us with hymns. In the spring, it was always "Easter Parade," and at Christmastime, "Rudolph the Red-Nosed Reindeer" and "Silent Night." His music filled many otherwise-silent gaps.

My parents divorced when I was 11. Even before then, my siblings and I had not enjoyed a close relationship with our father. He was remote, occasionally volatile, and often dismissive of children in general. He seemed truly happy only when he was playing his music.

Shortly after I turned 15, my father packed up my grandmother, whom we all adored, and moved to Arkansas. His absence brought a sense of relief. We already had what was, in effect, a long-distance relationship; geography was incidental. We couldn't have known then that Dad's move would lead to years of manipulation, guilt-trips, and fierce fighting over our not following him.

I don't think it's an understatement to say that, had it not been for our grandmother, the sweetest, gentlest woman I've ever known, we might not have seen Dad at all after they moved, especially during those first few years. But we loved her, so we relented. We kept our visits short and worked to forge some semblance of the closeness we longed for with him, but never quite managed to find. It just wasn't who he was.

The years stacked up, as years do. Our family celebrated high school and college graduations, weddings, and the births of grandchildren. Sometimes Dad would make it to the celebrations, sometimes he wouldn't. If there were any constants through those years, they would've been my dad's music, especially on everyone's birthday, when he made sure to call at the crack of dawn to play "Happy Birthday" to us on the organ, and his never-ending financial struggles. He called on us increasingly to bail him out.

***

We often wondered what would happen when our grandmother eventually passed away. But on a clear October night, Death surprised us all, taking not our grandmother, but our mother instead, at the age of 57. Suddenly, our father was the only parent we had left. This created a shift in our complicated relationship, a determination to hold on to our sole remaining parental connection, no matter how tenuous.

For a time after that, we enjoyed a period of relative "normalcy." This truce lasted for several years. But then our grandmother, who'd already passed 100 years of age, began to weaken. As her health deteriorated and our father's health began to falter, too, the old clashes stirred to life, with greater urgency now. There were renewed fights over Dad's convoluted finances, over how often we were able to visit, over our increasing concerns about whether he could safely care for our grandmother on his own anymore.

Once, when he tried to move her wheelchair up a curb to a restaurant, they both fell. Grandma sustained an awful-looking head wound, which a cousin who lived near them photographed and sent to us. Dad, in his effort to cushion her fall, had broken a rib and his glasses. On another occasion, Dad dropped Grandma in the church parking lot and was unable to lift her. Their pastor informed him, and us, they no longer wanted him to bring her to church on his own.

Even after he reluctantly accepted home visits from professional caregivers, we continued to receive reports from local cousins, neighbors, doctors, attorneys, caregivers, even some of Dad's friends, about hygiene issues, falls, minor car accidents, unpaid bills, overdrawn accounts, cut-off utilities, and threatened evictions. But, short of a court order and a protracted legal fight, because our father's doctor still considered him "competent," our hands were tied.

My three children, by now teens and a tween, began to dread the ringing of the phone. They knew that, at best, it meant their mom would be unavailable for homework help or advice or dinner; at worst, it meant she'd emerge from the office with red eyes and shoulders bowed with the weight of the latest report. Dad's savage refusals to accept the inevitabilities of his situation were taking an enormous toll on us all; sometimes, we'd take turns cutting off communications with him for a day or two. "I just can't talk to him this week, Jules," my older sister would say. "I just can't." A few days later, it'd be my turn.

By then, we adult children had all scattered among three different states, none of them Arkansas. With our children in school and jobs to hold down, we were facing what one might call a triple-decker of a generational sandwich, caring not only for an aging *parent* on one end and young kids on the other, but also the added layer of an elderly *grandparent*. With financial and family responsibilities of our own, we were not in a position to move to Arkansas to help; but Dad refused to move closer to any of us so we could help him. We had reached a devastating stalemate.

Finally, Dad and Grandma were formally evicted from their trailer home. We scrambled to find them an affordable, accessible apartment. The move took a toll on Dad's health, even as he continued to care for Grandma. Still, he continued to fight, telling us at one point that he had every intention of "going down" fighting.

***

Grandma held on a little longer. Dad cared for her until the last few weeks of her life, when he finally relented and allowed her to be admitted into a care facility. He stayed by her side every minute. Just before midnight on Christmas Eve, she slipped away at last. It's horrible to admit, but I felt relief along with my sorrow, even as we wondered what Dad would do next.

So soon after Grandma's death wasn't the time to press him; all his fight seemed to have left him, so once again, we stepped back. We called him often, made extra visits, continued to encourage him to move closer to us, but tried to give him the time and space he needed. He told us he was trying to get things organized back home, told us he was "fine." When you live so far away from someone, it's disturbingly easy to believe them when they say things like that.

***

Several months passed before we learned how far from fine Dad really was. We knew from the landlady's description, when she called my sister to notify us he was being evicted due to a "bug problem," that the condition of Dad's apartment would be pretty bad, but nothing—and I mean *nothing*—could've prepared us for what we saw when my dad opened his door that Sunday morning.

I didn't cry when I crossed the threshold into my father's filthy, overheated apartment and saw the hoarder's path he'd carved out of the mountains of newspapers and boxes, the heaps of old fast food containers littering the floor, and the mounds of mildewing clothes, both his and Grandma's, overflowing her two sitting chairs.

I didn't cry when I took my first—and last—breath through my nose. I didn't cry when I saw the cockroaches and the flies, covering every surface of the place, or the residue of their sticky excretions glistening on every wall and every cabinet—even on the keys of his beloved organ.

I didn't cry when I saw the sink full of rotting food, dirty dishes, and stagnant, greasy water. No, I didn't break, not until I opened the refrigerator and the freezer and found them both filled with bugs, dead bodies by the cupful and the living crawling in and out of bags of liquefied produce and putrid meats.

How could this have happened in just a few months?

I turned around and walked right back out to the parking lot, trying to breathe, trying not to vomit, wanting to run and never, ever look back. I stood behind my car, trying to come to grips with the awful situation that lay ahead of us; trying to find the strength to step back into that den of horrors; praying to God to fill me with the compassion I would need to see this task through, compassion for a broken man, my broken father, who'd been living in that unspeakable horror for *months*.

God must've heard my prayer, because somehow, we made it through that first unimaginable day, and the next, and the next. Dad—frail, unwashed, and bewildered— alternated between tears and anger, shame and gratitude, between dumpster-diving angrily behind our backs and apologizing for having let his life come to this.

The three of us—my sister, her husband, and I—tag-teamed him, distracting him and taking him out to eat at fast food places, directing his attention elsewhere as we made trip after trip to the apartment dumpster. When the awful job was finished, we threw away every piece of clothing we were wearing—even our shoes.

The next day, I got on a plane to head back to my husband and kids; my sister, brother-in-law, and Dad began the drive back to Illinois together. He'd agreed to move there with them. I hadn't spoken to my children at all during the trip. What could I possibly have said about what I was going through, about what their grandfather had been going through? Even now, months later, I struggle to find the right words.

Trauma, certainly. For weeks afterwards, every inch of my skin crawled 24/7; every speck on the floor or wall was evidence I'd brought his infestation into my own home. *Anger*, at my father's intractability and its awful cost. *Heartbreak*, at the loss of so many of my grandmother's things; with my own two hands, I'd pushed her wheelchair to the dumpster. Though they were just things, they were also a part of her—her aprons, her hats, her handwriting. All gone. *Fear*, over what the future holds for my dad, and for my sister and her family, who will bear the brunt of the responsibility for his care for the remainder of his days. *Shame*, that this would be the legacy my father would leave for my children.

Shame, too, that this is the legacy I *allowed* to become my father's.

***

It's the night after my return, and my husband and I have brought our daughter to the church for her chamber music concert. Though I'm still feeling sick and shaken from the past few days, I wouldn't miss it for anything. She's practiced for months on our old piano, an ancient Steinway my dad handed down to me years ago. I still remember him playing "Happy Birthday" to me on it in our garage the day he brought it up from Arkansas.

I sit now in the darkened church, feeling dirty and ashamed, until the opening notes rise up, washing over me. The choir joins in on my daughter's cue, and I begin to weep. As many times as I've heard her play the piece, which was inspired by the poem "There Will Be Rest," by Sara Teasdale, I've never heard the lyrics. I close my eyes, hearing the words for the first time, and the pain, the trauma, and the anger begin to subside.

The music and the message, the clarity and the peace, of these young voices, the power of my daughter's sure hands, they cleanse me, they bind up my wounds. I realize the meaning I needed to find is here, in the music soaring through the church, in the music that has always been love for my Dad, in the music that was, perhaps, the only way he knew how to express it.

I listen to these beautiful words, and I understand that it's up to me to decide what effect this pain will bear on my life. I think to myself, yes, I *will* make this world, even these last few days, of my own devising. I will focus not on my father's sickness and ruin, not on my shame and sadness, but, instead, on the truth of these words and the divinity of the music. This is my choice, to let the decades of hurt and betrayal and longing for my father's love wash away, leaving only the purity of compassion and love. My father's legacy will not be one of bankruptcy and failure, of mistakes and illness. I will devise, instead, *this* legacy, this gift of music, his music, this single, holy gift, passed down from my father, through me, to my daughter. It is a gift of perfect love.

Julia Tagliere is a freelance writer and editor and studied in the M.A. in Creative Writing program at DePaul University in Illinois. Her work has appeared in The Writer *and* Hay & Forage Grower *magazines, and she is a featured author for Buzzle, a content website. Julia's debut novel,* Widow Woman, *was published in 2012. In 2014, Open to Interpretation, the juried photography and prose series, selected Julia's short story, "The Navigator," for publication in* Love + Lust, *its fourth and final installment. Julia's latest story, "Te Absolvo," won Best Short Story in the 2015 William Faulkner Literary Competition. An active blogger and past finalist in Minneapolis' Loft Literary Center's Mentor Series Competition, Julia resides in Maryland with her family, where she is currently pursuing her M.A. in Fiction Writing at Johns Hopkins University*

THE THINGS YOU DO FOR LOVE
By Katherine Mikkelson

My dad read to us. I don't just mean when we were little, snuggled on the couch next to him, my brother and me struggling to sound out the words of *The Poky Little Puppy* (one of my all-time favorites) or *The Cat in the Hat*. No, my dad read to us long after we could read for ourselves, when we were tweens. Classics like *The Adventures of Tom Sawyer* and *Watership Down*. He was a master of dialogue and intonation, giving different voices to all of the characters, adding drama that could never be accomplished with a silent read. After we were a little older, "Reading by Dad" slowly fell away, a victim of overscheduled high schoolers who had to juggle sports and clubs and homework and friends. No one was more disappointed than my mom, who was always its most fervent champion.

Sometime after we became adults and moved away, "Reading By Dad" resumed with my dad reading to my mom. These days, when they visit, I can hear my dad's mellifluous voice from several rooms away, with my mom occasionally commenting, "Oh my!" or "I didn't see that coming." My dad so cheerfully obliges my mom that I was stunned when Dad recently confided to my husband that he doesn't particularly like reading out loud. He told my husband it makes it hard to follow the plot.

At first I was shocked and then I was confused. "Reading by Dad" is so synonymous with my father, it almost defines him. *Why did he spend all those years reading to us if he didn't enjoy it?* I wondered. And then it dawned on me—my dad read to us because he knew we all loved it and *that* brought him joy.

We all do this. Whether it's sitting with our mothers through chemo treatments or enduring a mommy-and-me art class with our toddlers, we do things we might not particularly enjoy, things that make us uncomfortable, things we might even dread, because they're important to those we love.

***

This was never more evident to me after hearing the saga of my friend—let's call her Sharon—and her mom, who suffers from mild dementia. About a year after Sharon moved her mother into a local assisted-care facility, Sharon's sister moved across the country for a new job. The sister began talking to Sharon about relocating their mom there as well. Sharon and the rest of the family agreed and plans were hatched to move Sharon's mom to another facility near the sister. Sharon then worked for several months to prepare her mom for a two-thousand mile, cross-country move.

All was well and good for a few months until Sharon learned her mom had moved in with a man she met at the facility. Sharon's sister thinks it's cute that her mom has a boyfriend; Sharon, not so much. She doesn't trust the guy. A significant age difference, a decision that is completely out of character for her mom, and her mom's compromised judgment, all worry Sharon. *What are this man's motives?* she wonders. *Could her mom be the potential victim of financial fraud?*

Despite her rapidly deteriorating memory, Sharon's mother *never* forgets her social security number. The woman may do things like leave her checkbook in the fridge, but her SSN is engraved on her brain like a tattoo which she proudly rattles off at the slightest provocation. *Would her mom rattle these important numbers without considering the implications?* Sharon worried. As if the general fears weren't enough, after googling her mom's new "boyfriend," Sharon learned he has a criminal record for—you guessed it—embezzlement.

Armed with this information, Sharon now looks out for her mom's financial health in addition to her physical and emotional health—ordering credit reports, requesting credit freezes, and carefully monitoring her mom's bank accounts. And through it all, Sharon's sister insists that Sharon shouldn't worry.

"Families are complicated," Sharon tells me when we

talk, painfully aware this was her mom's final move and that she won't be living nearby ever again. We continue our walk discussing how sometimes current resentments or past slights can hamper adult children from doing what's best for their parent. "I do all of this for mom because I want to stay connected," she says. Sharon doesn't enjoy ordering credit reports or biting her tongue, of course, but she does it because she loves her mom despite the tumult.

Another friend—let's call this friend Anne—absolutely detests musical theater. She finds it ridiculous that a character would suddenly break into song about finding love, squandering second chances, or not living up to one's potential. She would never willingly see *Les Miserables*, *My Fair Lady*, *The Sound of Music*, or any number of great stage productions and movies that've won countless awards. Despite this aversion, in a great twist of cosmic fate, Anne's two sons have been actively involved in musical theater for years. Her older son participated in high school drama club as an actor, and her younger son is currently on the tech crew. And, of course, Anne sucks it up and attends all these performances. "I absolutely dread the shows," she told me. "But I always leave with so much admiration. I'm just fascinated that my boys run eagerly into the spotlight. I don't get it or understand it or like it, but I love watching them love it."

I, too, have found myself stuck in the middle, trying

to please both parent and child, doing activities I'd hardly choose on my own—but I do them because they're important to those I love. My younger son fenced for years in both elementary school and middle school. Despite the countless times he explained the rules and the scoring to me, I could barely tell the difference between a parry and a passé, a foil and epee—the two styles of fencing weaponry—and constantly confused the target areas.

My lack of knowledge and understanding of the sport made it difficult to watch his tournaments. I never knew what was happening and when he removed his face mask, I was met with tears, anger, or elation, none of which I could anticipate. Additionally, fencing, like many competitive sports, is often an all-day or multiple-day affair with lots of waiting around, interspersed with moments of sheer terror when your kid is the one competing. Such long days, and so much waiting around until the nervous energy coalesces and erupts like a long dormant volcano. On top of this, the expensive equipment and travel costs made it feel like money was flying out of my wallet during my son's tenure as a fencer.

But while I didn't love fencing, I loved every minute of watching my son love fencing.

Just like I love watching my mother love gardens. She has always been fascinated with botanical gardens, and at her request, I've visited more botanical gardens than

I can remember: from Winterthur Museum and Gardens in Delaware, to Butchart Gardens in Victoria, British Columbia, and even a few gardens overseas. One time, the quest to find Retreat Gardens in Nassau in the Bahamas led us on a hike all over the island to a—shall we say—non-touristy area where the locals gave us the side-eye for invading their neighborhood. A kind woman stopped her car and gently urged us to go back to our hotel. Yet despite all this traipsing around in search of and through the gardens, do I know vaccinium from vinca? Nope, I do not. Do I relish blooming begonias or containers of cosmos? Not one bit. But I visit these gardens for her, because Mom is the type of person who gets excited when she sees the rare silversword in bloom and that excitement makes me smile.

***

I'm all too aware that our time with parents and children is finite. We have to embrace the not-so-fun along with the fun because before we know it, children grow up and move out, and parents become old and infirm. So we hold Dad's arm a little tighter when we walk him out of the senior center, as he curses after losing again in his weekly bridge game. We bite our tongue when our daughter flinches and complains as we pin up her hair before her ballet recital where she will most assuredly forget a few steps. And we savor the drops from each less-than-enjoyable moment because you never know when they'll evaporate. And when they do, we can savor them no more.

Katherine Mikkelson is a recovering attorney turned writer. She writes a food blog at stateeats.com. and her work has appeared in Adoptive Families Magazine *and the* Chicago Tribune. *An essay, "Purple Fleece and Motherhood" appeared in the anthology,* Not What I Expected: The Unpredictable Road From Womanhood to Motherhood *(Paycock Press, 2007). She lives in the Chicago area with her husband, Tom, and is the mother of two boys.*

GETTING TO KNOW DAD
By Diana Walters

Betty, my stepmother, called to tell me my father was having heart problems and would be going in for tests. We talked about the details for a few minutes before she added, "Diana, something else is going on with your dad. He's acting different. For one thing, he's spending money on crazy things. Last week he bought a Buick! We don't need a new car, and we can't afford it. I talked him into taking it back, but he was furious. The checkbook is a mess. I have no idea how much money is in there. He doesn't like me looking at it."

I thought she was overreacting. Dad's behavior had always been unpredictable. Although he'd been conservative with money, he'd also prided himself on his ability to "wheel and deal." I remembered all the items he bought, sold, and traded when I was growing up. Tools, musical instruments, and various household appliances would come and go. One time, he negotiated for the purchase of a child-size train that ran on a track in our backyard, although before long it was replaced with a backhoe.

As for his anger, he'd never been a warm, loving person. Maybe he and Betty had been married long enough for her to see what kind of man he really was. His moods erratic, he was a formidable presence in my childhood. My siblings and I were, in fact, still intimidated by him, although we were adults with children of our own.

Dad had been quick to criticize our smallest infraction when we were kids. There was no way to please him. He yelled at times, but he didn't have to raise his voice to command our attention. Still, I craved his affection.

Before bed every night, after kissing my mom and receiving her "I love you," I'd turn and kiss my dad's cheek and say, "Goodnight, I love you Dad." And, in return, he'd simply grunt. This ritual exasperated my sister. "Why do you bother?" she'd ask. "How can you stand to be ignored night after night? He's never going to say it back you know." Eventually, I too, gave up.

***

I married at nineteen, left home, and raised a family. The years passed, and I maintained a polite, although distant, relationship with my father. On the rare occasions we came together as a family, I viewed Dad as the domineering, critical parent of our youth. I often felt like a child again in his presence. For the most part, I avoided the sting of his criticism by staying away. I dutifully called each week, usually talking to Betty, but although I lived only a half-hour's drive from them, I seldom visited.

But now he was having heart problems, and I felt an

urgency to spend time with him before it was too late. I decided I'd meet him on neutral ground—the mall where he and Betty walked each day. He wouldn't shout or argue with me in public. It was a safe place to get reacquainted.

In spite of health issues and pain in his legs, Dad insisted on walking the perimeter of the mall two times each day. "Use it or lose it," he'd say. Afterward, he sat in the coffee shop drinking cup after cup of decaf while Betty shopped. That's where I began looking for him two or three times a week.

The first time I showed up, Dad was surprised but seemed pleased to see me. Our conversations were stilted at first as I tentatively tried to build a new relationship. I didn't know what to say to him, feeling certain he'd criticize me again if I said the wrong thing. However, I found that instead of criticism, Dad's conversation often turned philosophical and reflective. He no longer seemed like the opinionated, domineering personality of my youth. He actually asked me about my life and seemed interested in the answer. One day he commented that he'd not been a good father. "I shouldn't have treated you kids that way."

I discovered that my dad had a sense of humor. I didn't remember much laughter around the house when I was growing up, but now he laughed easily and heartily. It became my mission to prepare a story or joke to entertain him. Much to my surprise, I began to enjoy the time we spent together.

I didn't notice immediately that humor was a way for him to cover up lapses in memory. He never gave direct answers to my questions. "Dad, I don't remember, did you finish tenth grade or eleventh?"

"Doesn't matter. I learned everything I needed to know on the dance floor," he chuckled. And queries about my childhood were met with, "You ought to know, you were there." Little by little, his memory deficit became more pronounced, especially his short-term memory. He'd ask, "Where's Betty?" I'd answer that she went shopping and would be back soon. Fifteen minutes later, "Where's Betty?"

Over the next year, he became increasingly confused. He was diagnosed with vascular dementia. Then, he started needing help with his personal care. When Betty wasn't able to take Dad to the mall or leave him home alone any more, I stayed with him while she grocery shopped. Dad could carry on a conversation, although he often repeated himself, and his memory loss was sometimes heartrending. For example, he'd often forget my mother was dead. "Where's Nell?" he'd ask. I'd remind him she was in heaven and that he was married to Betty now. One time he asked if his brother Lloyd had died. I said, "Yes." He asked about his younger brother. "What about Bill?

Is he alive?" When I replied honestly, he shook his head sadly. "They're all gone," he said.

He still had a sense of humor, though, and I could make him laugh with exaggerated stories about people I knew. He laughed at himself as well. Dad often forgot he could no longer walk. When I wasn't looking, he'd struggle to his feet and immediately slide to the floor in a heap. Mercifully, he never got hurt. He would quip, "My round body bounces like a rubber ball."

One weekend, Betty went out of town to visit her sister who was ill. Dad was bed bound by then and needed total care. Although we had a caregiver coming to help me several hours each day, I needed to change his Depend underwear before she arrived. In spite of his confusion, Dad knew it was not proper for a daughter to see her father undressed. He pushed me away and growled "get away from there." It took some convincing—and some lying—before he allowed me to care for him. I told him I was a trained caregiver, I was like a nurse, and I took care of men all the time.

Soon after that, Dad wouldn't be able to communicate in words, but I was grateful for the hours I had with him, laughing, talking, and getting to know the person he'd become. In spite of the dementia, we made some new memories, good ones this time.

When Betty returned from visiting her sister, I was

2

48 | *Here In The Middle: Stories of Love, Loss, and Connection*

exhausted and eager to get home to my husband and my usual routine. Dad had been dozing off most of the day, and I considered leaving without saying goodbye. Instead, I bent over him and whispered, "Goodnight Dad. I'll see you soon. I love you."

Dad opened his eyes. Ever so slowly, he raised his hand and patted my cheek. His voice was weak, but I heard as clearly as if he'd shouted the words: "Love you, too."

Diana Walters is the manager of an assisted living unit in Chattanooga, Tennessee, and a freelance writer. She and her husband develop materials and provide training for ministry to people with dementia. Her original research was published in Dementia: The International Journal of Social Research and Practice. Her devotionals have been published in The Upper Room and Oblates.

FRAGILE
By Caroline M. Grant

My son Eli likes to cook. In kindergarten he invented a cake—a chewy, chocolate chip sheet cake, softened with milk and sweetened with honey—that's become a staple in our family, and then he followed it up with a couple cookie recipes, riffs on classic chocolate chip and peanut butter.

Now a third grader, he's standing at the stove scrambling eggs just like his dad taught him. He sets the pan on the flame and adds a pat of butter, then goes to the cupboard for a bowl and to the fridge for an egg. By the time he circles back to the stove, the butter is melted; he lifts the pan and tips it in a slow swirl, then sets it gently down, cracks his egg into the bowl, and gives it a little scramble before pouring it slowly into the pan. I love watching him, love every aspect of this scene: that he learned from his dad; that he's cooking his own breakfast; that he approaches it all with such care.

But it doesn't last. "I don't like cracking eggs," he admits. "It's too messy." He doesn't like the unpredictability of the crack. You tap an egg against the counter, but where exactly will it break, and how big a crack will form? Will the egg come spilling right out? Will it bring fragments of shell with it? Will the membrane catch and hold inside? He likes order and routine and control. The best thing is what happened before. The best meal is one he's already eaten.

Am I a good mother for him because I feel the same way? Or should I push harder for us both? Eggs are a challenge. We go a while longer with me cracking the eggs for him, but then he abandons them for cold cereal, avocado toast, an apple sliced and spread with almond butter—assembling, not cooking.

Not that I'm in any position to judge. My kids do homework while I start dinner; I pause as Eli tells me what the pharaohs took to their geometric graves, then again to glance at my e-mail; there's one from Dad looking for recipes, frustrated with my mom's shrinking appetite and unpredictable palate. His worry seems to rise from my phone like steam and then I realize, *Oh!* The rice has boiled over and the vegetables are shriveling in a dry, burning pan. My husband puts his hands on my shoulders and moves me away from the stove; I e-mail my dad some pasta ideas and book a flight east to cook and pack for my parents.

Soon, they'll move from the house they built in rural Connecticut into an assisted living residence near my family in San Francisco. Everything about this transition feels *correct*—they made the plan, acknowledging Mom's declining health; they're strong enough to make the move; they liked two of the twelve communities I scouted for them and made their own decision—but it doesn't yet feel *good*.

I'll miss their house, despite its population of uninvited mice and ladybugs. I'll miss clumps of daffodils blooming against gray stone walls in the spring and fallen leaves frozen into the pond in winter. I'll miss watching my boys walk down to the garden or orchard with their granddad and guessing what they'll carry back to the kitchen: sweet, knobby apples; red potatoes with clumps of dirt still clinging; small green heads of broccoli with the occasional pale worm curled in its florets.

***

But once I arrive, I stop my sad reminiscing and focus. I cook and stock my parents' freezer. I sort, pack, and label. I drive loads to Goodwill (a forty-five-minute drive), to the hospital consignment shop (twenty minutes), and to the library (fifteen). I set some things aside for an auction house, some for my siblings, and others for cousins. I winnow my mom's entire book collection in one evening; behind one shelf, I find a mouse has stored his winter's supply of acorns. *Sorry, mouse*, I think as I sweep his pantry into the trash.

Then it's back to the kitchen, where I fill containers with lasagna and casserole and soup, but mostly I beat eggs into endless quiches, soft and easy to eat, stuffed with vegetables from Dad's garden and poured into whole wheat crusts rolled out with Mom's old maple rolling pin, its red-painted handles faded from years of use. I'm going for quantity and freezability here; the cooking feels utilitarian, purposeful. I wrap, label, stack, and then close the freezer on more than a dozen meals.

I consider the cliché—you have to break a few eggs to make an omelette—in light of my son and my parents. Eli would've preferred to scramble without any cracking and so, too, would I prefer to pull off my parents' move without any fuss or mess. Just float them out to San Francisco and present them with their new home: smaller, but with their same pineapple-stenciled curtains; those old familiar curtains, a story in themselves for me to clean, press, tailor, flameproof (with certification from the fire department inspector), and rehang on newly installed hardware. Instead of a dirt road and maple trees, the curtains frame a view of busy 19th Avenue and, if you stretch up on tiptoes and the fog has cleared, a glimpse of the Golden Gate Bridge.

I hire someone to help sort, donate, pack, and finally ship the things my parents want in San Francisco, but she, too, is preoccupied by her aging parents and can't give this job her full, professional attention. She and I e-mail back and forth, exchanging lists and spreadsheets, but still things fall through the cracks. Literally. Glasses are broken. A set of twelve Japanese plates—all I really craved from my parents' things—arrives, missing three, and I cry as I unpack, searching through the box, knowing it's empty but still hoping maybe somehow this last crumple of tissue paper will solidify into pottery. My priorities are foolish, I know; my parents are fine, and when Mom walks through the door, she says, "It looks like home." I exhale for the first time, it feels, in months.

A few days later, leaving their new apartment after a visit, I start down the hall and pause, disoriented. A faint institutional whiff of carpet cleaner and canned pears hits me powerfully and makes me homesick for my parents, even though they're just steps away. I make it down to the car and drive home, but I can't shake the odd feeling. As I fall asleep that night, my back hurts and I think I've strained it lifting boxes.

I'm woken by my ribs cinching tight, my breathing constricted and my heart racing. I climb out of bed trying to leave the feeling behind, only to fall to my knees in a faint. My husband, alarmed, helps me up and back into bed where I sob and gasp. Eventually my heartbeat slows. I can breathe. I can sleep. In the morning, I consult Dr. Google and realize I've had a panic attack. In my sleep? This seems absurd and cruel. How unfair that the stress simmering beneath the thin shell of my skin can bubble up and grip me so hard.

But then it happens again. I'm driving Dad across the new Bay Bridge, remarking on the structure's gleaming white cables, the roadway low on the water, when I feel it all fall away beneath me. My hands clench the steering wheel to keep afloat. Dad doesn't notice my pinched tone and grip, and once we're off the bridge I exhale. And then a third time, at the cathedral for evensong, I glance up the nave and the soaring tower dizzies me. I tilt my head down, eyes closed as if in prayer, no one close enough to see that my hands are holding tight to the edge of the pew so that I don't fall.

***

Mom and Dad have now lived here a year. Their house and land in Connecticut sold. We're planning a vacation together. I drive them to the gerontologist, the eye doctor, the hearing-aid specialist, the neurologist, the memory and aging clinic, the physical therapist, for blood work, a flu shot, an MRI, an EEG. I take them to church and then bring them to my house for lunch afterward. I can cook differently for them here, fresh meals that don't need to survive the freezer, but it's often still a familiar quiche on the menu.

One morning I arrive to take Mom to physical therapy and wait and wait. This is a routine that's become routine: twice a week, 9:45 a.m. I hesitate to call, afraid the phone will ring just as she's walking out the door and that she could trip and fall in her rush to answer it. I hesitate to head upstairs, afraid I'll miss her coming down the elevator. The minutes tick by—now we'll certainly be late—and I decide to race up. She forgot about the appointment, but she readies herself deliberately while I call the therapist. I know we don't need to rush—certainly these patients are late all the time—but I can't help myself.

On the drive, I will the stoplights to green, will the pedestrians to cross more quickly, will the driver backing carefully out of the parking space to make way for me. Taking Mom by the elbow, I guide her from the car to the entrance, paying more attention to her footing than to my own, and slam my head into a low tree branch. I reel, catch my balance, never letting go of Mom. The physical therapist greets me with concern, fetches an ice pack, and I can't catch her eye lest the tears brimming in my eyes overflow. "I'm okay," I signal with a nod. "I'll be okay."

After Mom's appointment, my head throbbing, I struggle to hold it together while I drive her home. She reaches out and touches my shoulder. "Oh, Caroline," she murmurs. "I'm sorry. I'm so sorry." How long has it been since she's had a chance to mother me? We continue without speaking, her hand on my shoulder, comforting me.

I think of all the things I'd like to control—mom's

aging, my schedule, Eli's cooking (my cooking!), our health, our lives—and the list unfurls like a dropped ball of yarn, rolling out of reach. But sitting in the car with Mom, I start to feel a shift in perspective, as if the crack on the head has shaken something loose in me. I'm not Zen enough to let it all go; I'd still like less mess. But it's a start. And when I get home, I call out to Eli and we cook some eggs.

Caroline M. Grant is the co-director of the Sustainable Arts Foundation. She served on the editorial board of Literary Mama for ten years, including five as editor-in-chief, and has also co-edited two anthologies: The Cassoulet Saved Our Marriage: True Tales of Food, Family, and How We Learn to Eat *(Roost Books, 2013) and* Mama, PhD: Women Write About Motherhood and Academic Life *(Rutgers University Press, 2008). She lives in San Francisco with her husband and two sons.*

THEY GROW OLD SO FAST
By Jennie Robertson

Grammie gingerly walks the snowy path towards her big yellow farmhouse, unaided by even a cane at the age of 93. I follow closely behind, arms extended just enough to be ready to catch her, though I've never needed to—someday I might need to, someday soon. Her soft, fuzzy white head reaches just about to my shoulder, and I'm only five feet tall—Grammie is now a tiny person. I wonder how tall she was before she started getting shorter. I wonder at what point we passed each other.

I spend the day writing at her long kitchen table, tapping into the energy and rhythm of the thousand mornings she spent kneading her sorrows into joy and her dough into bread on its wooden surface. At my back is the black, cast-iron, Glenwood cook stove that anchors all my ideas of home. I've spent many days in my life this way, and, truth be told, I'm glad to be doing it again, even though it's because we can't leave her alone, lest she fall or burn the house down or fall prey to unscrupulous overcharging "handymen." When I was tiny, I spent the days watching TV in Grammie's living room while she worked in the kitchen, occasionally peeking in at me. Now our roles have reversed.

I spent every day of my early childhood at Grammie's house while my mother taught school. I don't have memories of her sitting down during the day; she gardened, she cooked, she tackled laundry and home repairs. Sometimes she hired my cousins and siblings and me to do these repairs. She inspired an enviable work ethic that I value and wish I had the backbone to instill in the kids I occasionally hire. She didn't pay for shoddy or unfinished work. When my cousin came in for lunch one day and lingered a bit too long, she gave him a sharp but affectionate look and said he might as well get back to work because there wasn't any dessert.

In her home, I learned to associate work with happiness, love, and fulfillment. My cousins and I begged to be allowed to muck out the pony; we raced to pile firewood on the wheeled cart and heave it inside; we washed dishes together after many merry dinners, singing, laughing.

My hard-working Grammie has earned her rest, which she now takes most of the day in her recliner, although occasionally we find some beans for her to snap or peas to shell; she cheerfully obliges. She snoozes a lot, though she claims she "never naps." She opens a novel and reads wherever her eyes land. She embroiders; we even convinced her to enter a piece in the fair this year, and she won a ribbon. My children and my sister's children play beside her, and often I look up to see them piled on her lap, three or four deep, listening to her read them a story. She can't always name all of them or remember whose child is whose, but she knows they're her great-grandchildren and has plenty of affection for them, and they for her.

She was past 90 when she stopped getting down on the floor at their urging; I'm not sure she has stopped, in fact. There's no ignoring the fact that the list of things she does is getting shorter, though; last year at this time, she made me lunch when I was there. Now I make it, trying to cook the old favorites she taught me, trying to tempt her finicky appetite. If red flannel hash won't do it, maybe fish chowder will, or chipped beef on toast. There are many other little tasks besides cooking that she has slowly, silently stopped performing—hanging out the laundry, sweeping the floor. It's hard to find something to take their place.

***

Sometimes I look at her and hope to age as well as she has, though I won't, since I didn't spend the first or any years of my life in a healthy, if desperate, Depression-era cycle of eating garden food I labored to grow myself. Sometimes, though, I look at her and hope I don't live as long, such as when her last surviving sibling died this past year, several years past her hundredth birthday. Everyone she loved hasn't gone—we're still here. But so many have. Her husband, my grandfather, died thirty years ago. I imagine outliving my husband by thirty years and decide, guiltily, to have another artery clogging cookie. But then I look at my children and imagine reading to their grandchildren when I'm 90. I start my diet again.

I guess everyone knows about the excruciating pain of watching your loved ones age and fade away and the awkward possibilities when caring for aging bodies. What I didn't know or expect is the acute tenderness that is heavy but still joyful; it squeezes my heart unbidden at odd moments. It's similar to what I feel for a child, protective and affectionate; but then again, it's different, too, etched with history, enriched with earned respect. A child is like a blank book, smooth, full of sweet possibilities, unblemished. Grammie is a tale that is almost told, bound in exquisite leather with a worn patina, a revered book that opens to the best-loved parts. Fragile, but full of wisdom. Weighty, but worth the effort.

Everyone tells you to treasure the small moments with your children, but not many mention the fleeting years at the other end of life. The days are long, as they say, investing so many hours in Grammie's care, but the years are short, and, unlike with children, there is only a sweet memory waiting at the end. This is my reminder to myself: Enjoy the grilled cheese sandwiches at Grammie's big kitchen table. Listen to her sing while she peels the supper potatoes. Tell her again, patiently, every time she asks what the plan is for the day, or the hour. This season is precious. They grow old so fast.

In loving memory
Sophie Elizabeth Hurd
February 1921-August 2016

Jennie Robertson lives and writes in her native state of Maine. She's been published in Mary Jane's Farm, Mothers Always Write, Literary Mama, and the HerStories anthology, So Glad They Told Me. *She is a regular contributor to Thinking Outside the Sandbox.*

THE SPACE BETWEEN
By Linda A. Janssen

I can't recall the precise moment when I officially became a member of the Sandwich Generation, caught squarely between the extraordinary needs of parent and child. I didn't awaken one morning with the letter 'S' tattooed on my forehead or receive a welcome letter from the local chapter of Sandwiched Generation, International. I came to realize something had shifted, something I couldn't rationalize or control or bargain my way out of. Membership in this unwelcome association never falters, as new pledges arrive on the threshold of this uncertain terrain and weary graduates retreat.

I'm not talking about the hazy period of months and years during which the decline of aging parents pushes aside our denial and a new reality slowly comes into focus. Nor do I mean the usual growing pains of raising children: the demands of infancy, the unpredictability of toddlerhood, the awkwardness of pre- and early-adolescence, or the more nuanced challenges of the teen years. It isn't about the pressures of work, career, giving back, finding yourself, or finding your way.

What I'm referring to is the dawning recognition that we're suddenly pulled between non-negotiable needs of two or more loved ones. *Life must change*. It's no longer a case of making suggestions, giving guidance, and helping out. Instead, it's now a matter of stepping in, taking over, making decisions, and bearing responsibility for what results. It's a reordering of our world, pushing aside much of what we've always thought of as "must do's," and shrinking this life list down to only the essential elements. It's being between the proverbial rock and a hard place, not for a short, uncomfortable period of time, but for an enduring, painful near and not-so-near future. It's excruciating, entering this battlefield of crisis. We don't simply survive; we're redefined.

***

For my immediate family, it was a child's diagnosis of a medical condition at the same time my father was dying of pancreatic cancer. My mother, in addition to experiencing grief and not-unexpected situational depression, was also showing signs of dementia. After my father's death, it seemed at first we could support my mother and our child in a tag-team manner, rushing from one to the other, addressing immediate needs and weathering crises as they cropped up. In between episodes in what has proved to be a long-running sequence, we'd collapse in exhaustion, rest up and then survey the landscape, desperate to discern what was ahead. Over time, we found that ping-ponging between the two for emergencies or setbacks had given way to juggling both at the same time.

The specifics of this "sandwiching" in our family are not important; everyone in the throes of this will deal with different details, but a number of constants remain. It's a cauldron of the worst sort, watching as the ones who gave life to you and to whom you have given life struggle. You endure the pain of observing their pain. Secretly you may rant and rail and thrash and scream, but eventually you realize—both far too soon and far too late—that doing so doesn't change a thing and isn't worth the exertion. Conservation of energy becomes top of mind. Some days, the only thing that keeps you going is the knowledge that if you falter, your child or your parent (or sadly, both) suffers more for the lack of your presence and your actions.

For me, the past few years have meant a clearing of the decks: professional goals, personal aspirations, socializing, certain friendships, energetic endeavors, sometimes even my cherished writing, have all been swept aside. What has remained is a hunkering down, a safeguarding of attention, energy and effort saved for only the most necessary of actions to help, to heal, or to hold space for the inevitable.

I've learned to say "no" to the unnecessary or to someone else's priority which doesn't rise to the level of my own, and "yes" to that which provides some measure of relief to any aspect of our situation or sustenance to the soul. For everything else, I've learned to ditch the waffling non-response of a maybe, answering instead with a firm "I'll give that careful thought and get back to you." I have learned to be specific when asking for what's needed and helpful in the most difficult times, and as a result, have experienced firsthand the appreciation others feel when they, too, can contribute and otherwise lighten the load.

When I first heard the term "Sandwich Generation," I visualized just that: a baguette or roll, some chicken or cheese, perhaps tomato, lettuce, and preferred condiment of choice. Now when I hear it, I see that rock and that hard place, wedged up next to each other with a scarcity of daylight between the two.

I know these mammoth slabs will not last forever: modern science, medical treatments, and the right prescriptions have made a world of difference both for healing our child and for easing my mother's retreat into herself. Continued progress and the passage of time have allowed the one to flourish and grow, while mortality beckons as the other withers and fades. Their situations are different, yet the weight bears down similarly.

In the meantime, I've learned there's space, room between the rock and the hard place, albeit deep and narrow and limited. These gaps, these cracks, these chasms grow and diminish as either the rock or the hard place expands and contracts. It's into these openings—

this space between—we learn to pour the rest of our lives, fitting in the moments of joy and laughter, faith and remembrance. It's into these fissures we place celebration and growth and renewal.

There are limited benefits to speak of, found primarily in retrospect. Hindsight is more than panning for the obvious nuggets of lessons learned. Rather, it's a gleaning of the tiniest kernels of truth, recognition, and understanding—hard-won from experience we neither desired nor requested. It's in the sifting of these seeds we come to recognize the intangible gifts received: the peace which comes from doing what we know to be right, the gradual replenishment of resilience depleted, a sense of what truly matters, and the healing power of abiding love.

Linda A. Janssen lives in Chapel Hill, NC, where she writes short stories, personal essays, creative nonfiction and the proverbial novel work-in-progress. Having lived in four countries and traveled to forty more, she loves exploring other cultures as much as characters. She is the author of the nonfiction book The Emotionally Resilient Expat: Engage, Adapt and Thrive Across Cultures (UK expatriate press Summertime Publishing, 2013), and has contributed to three other books on cross-cultural life. Linda also serves as the North Carolina Writers Network regional representative for Orange County.